Arroyo Center Center for Military Health Policy Research

Evaluation of the Low Back Pain Practice Guideline Implementation in the Army Medical Department

Donna O. Farley

Georges Vernez

Will Nicholas

Elaine S. Quiter

George J. Dydek

Suzanne Pieklik

Shan Cretin

Prepared for the United States Army
Approved for public release; distribution unlimited

RAND

The research described in this report was sponsored by the United States Army under Contract No. DASW01-01-C-0003.

Library of Congress Cataloging-in-Publication Data

Evaluation of the Low Back Pain Practice Guideline Implementation in the Army Medical Department / Donna Farley ... [et al.].
p. cm.
"MR-1758."
Includes bibliographical references.
ISBN 0-8330-3474-X (Paperback)
1. Backache—Treatment—Evaluation. I. Farley, Donna.

RD771.B217E94 2003
355.3'45'0973—dc22

2003020092

The RAND Corporation is a nonprofit research organization providing objective analysis and effective solutions that address the challenges facing the public and private sectors around the world. RAND's publications do not necessarily reflect the opinions of its research clients and sponsors.

Published 2004 by the RAND Corporation
1700 Main Street, P.O. Box 2138, Santa Monica, CA 90407-2138
1200 South Hayes Street, Arlington, VA 22202-5050
201 North Craig Street, Suite 202, Pittsburgh, PA 15213-1516
RAND URL: http://www.rand.org/
To order RAND documents or to obtain additional information, contact
Distribution Services: Telephone: (310) 451-7002;
Fax: (310) 451-6915; Email: order@rand.org

PREFACE

The RAND Corporation has been working with the Army Medical Department on a project entitled "Implementing Clinical Practice Guidelines in the Army Medical System." This project assisted the Army Medical Department in developing and testing methods to effectively implement clinical practice guidelines in the Army treatment facilities to achieve consistent and quality clinical care practices across the Army health system. Three sequential demonstrations were conducted to test and refine implementation methods before embarking on full implementation of practice guidelines across the Army health system. The three guidelines were those for primary care management of low back pain, asthma, and diabetes.

This report presents the final results of the evaluation that RAND conducted as part of the demonstration for the practice guideline for low back pain, which was conducted in 1999 and 2000. The evaluation included both (1) a process evaluation of the experiences of the participating military treatment facilities and (2) a quantitative evaluation to assess effects on processes of care associated with the introduction of best practices recommended by the practice guideline. In this report, we present and synthesize the findings from these two evaluation components with the goal of providing as complete a picture as possible of variations across facilities in relevant practices, the extent to which the demonstration sites changed their practices, and measurable effects these actions had on utilization of services and medications. This report is the first of three final reports being generated in this project. It will be followed by similar reports from the demonstrations for the asthma and diabetes practice guidelines. This report will be of interest to personnel in the military health services as well as to other organizations pursuing strategies for implementing best practices.

This research was sponsored by the U.S. Army Surgeon General. It was conducted jointly in the Manpower and Training Program of the RAND Arroyo Center, a federally funded research and development center sponsored by the United States Army, and in RAND Health's Center for Military Health Policy Research. RAND Arroyo Center and RAND Health's Center for Military Health Policy Research are part of the RAND Corporation.

For more information on RAND Arroyo Center, contact the Director of Operations (telephone 310-393-0411, extension 6419; FAX 310-451-6952; e-mail Marcy_Agmon@rand.org), or visit the Arroyo Center's Web site at http://www.rand.org/ard/.

CONTENTS

FIGURES

TABLES

SUMMARY

The Army Medical Department (AMEDD) is committed to establishing a structure and process to support its military/medical treatment facilities (MTFs) in implementing evidence-based practice guidelines to achieve best practices that reduce variation and enhance quality of medical care. AMEDD contracted with RAND to work as a partner in the development and testing of guideline implementation methods for ultimate application in an Army-wide guideline program. Taking the approach of testing new methods on a small scale, the AMEDD/RAND project fielded three sequential demonstrations over a two-year period, in each of which participating MTFs implemented a different clinical practice guideline. All the demonstrations worked with practice guidelines that were established collaboratively by the Departments of Veterans Affairs (VA) and Defense (DoD). In the first demonstration, four MTFs in the Great Plains Region implemented the practice guideline for low back pain. Next, the practice guideline for asthma was implemented by four MTFs in the Southeast Region. Last, the practice guideline for diabetes was implemented by two MTFs in the Western Region.

RAND performed evaluations for each demonstration that included a process evaluation and an analysis of effects on clinical practices. This report presents the findings from our evaluation of the implementation of the practice guideline for low back pain in the Great Plains Region demonstration. These findings incorporate and extend our earlier process evaluation findings for activities and progress during the first three months the demonstration MTFs worked with the low back pain demonstration.[1]

Specific components of RAND's evaluation for each demonstration included the following:

- *Process evaluation* documented the implementation activities of participating MTFs, described their successes in changing clinical practices, identified successes and challenges reported by the sites, and obtained their feedback regarding U.S. Army Medical Command (MEDCOM) support.
- *Analysis of effects* estimated the extent to which the sites' implementation activities affected specific measures of service delivery for low back pain, with comparisons to a control group of MTFs that did not implement the guideline.
- *Benchmarking* described variations in practices across MTFs for the measures used in the analysis of effects to help identify priorities for future interventions and for comparing individual facilities to benchmarks for target levels of performance.
- *Methods development* documented the measurement methods developed and the related data requirements to provide a basis for future systemwide monitoring of progress in achieving best practices for each condition addressed by a guideline.

BACKGROUND

DoD and the VA initiated a collaborative project in early 1998 to establish a single standard of care in the military and VA health systems, with the goals of (1) adaptation of existing clinical practice guidelines for selected conditions, (2) selection of two to four indicators for each guideline to benchmark and monitor implementation progress, and (3) integration of DoD/VA prevention, pharmaceutical, and clinical information efforts. With this approach to guideline development, DoD and the VA made a commitment to use of evidence-based practices in their health care facilities. Each practice guideline

---

[1] Unpublished RAND research by Donna O. Farley, Georges Vernez, Elaine S. Quiter, and Shan Cretin.

is a statement of best practices for the management and treatment of the health condition it addresses. The DoD/VA working group designated an expert panel to develop each practice guideline and to develop recommendations for the metrics to be used by the military services and the VA to monitor progress in guideline implementation. The recommendations for practices in each component of care take into account the strength of relevant scientific evidence, which is documented in the written practice guideline (VHA/DoD, 1999).

The Practice Guideline for Low Back Pain

The principal emphasis of the DoD/VA low back pain practice guideline is on acute low back pain, which is defined as low back pain occurring during the first six weeks after the initial onset of pain. Five key guideline elements were identified by the expert panel responsible for the low back pain guideline (see Chapter One, Table 1.1). The guideline recommends use of conservative treatment (minimal clinical intervention) for acute low back pain patients to allow recovery to take place naturally, which occurs in 80–90 percent of the patients. Patients should be educated on self-care management techniques, including reduction in activity and light exercises to help ease the pain. Imaging studies or laboratory tests are not recommended initially except for cases with symptoms indicating the presence of a more serious condition. Pain medications may be used to ease patients' discomfort, but these should not include muscle relaxants. The last part of the guideline addresses care for chronic low back pain, recommending referrals to physical therapy or manipulation for patients who do not respond to conservative treatment and have intense, continuing pain.

Expected Effects on Health Care Practices

When the MTFs implemented the low back pain guideline, clinical practices should have changed to reflect a new emphasis on conservative treatment for patients during the first six weeks following the initial visit (defined as acute low back pain), to be followed in later weeks by appropriate consultation and referral to specialists for patients who still have low back pain (defined by the guideline as chronic low back pain).[2] To the extent that MTFs had been treating acute low back pain patients more aggressively than the guideline recommends, we would expect reductions in the use of manipulation (by physical therapy or chiropractic), frequency of primary care visits, specialty referrals, imaging studies, laboratory tests, and prescriptions for pain medications during the first six weeks of care. For chronic low back pain patients, the use of specialty care and diagnostic tests was predicted to increase because the guideline offers direction to primary care providers that could encourage them to treat these patients more proactively than they had previously.

Our analyses focused on patterns of service delivery and pain medication prescriptions during the conservative treatment period. We tested six hypotheses, stating that increased use of conservative treatment for acute low back pain patients will lead to a decrease during the first six weeks of care in the

1. percentage of patients referred to physical therapy or manipulation
2. number of follow-up visits per low back pain patient
3. percentage of acute low back pain patients referred to specialty care
4. percentage of acute low back pain patients prescribed muscle relaxants
5. percentage of acute low back pain patients prescribed narcotics
6. percentage of nonsteroidal anti-inflammatory drugs (NSAIDs) prescribed that are high cost.

These hypotheses are based on the assumption that an MTF effectively introduces and maintains the new approach of conservative treatment, which involves reducing the amount of services and medications provided to patients during the early weeks of low back pain. Therefore, we expect to observe the hypothesized changes in clinical practices only in those MTFs that proactively implemented

[2]The guideline leaves the actual timing of specialty referrals to the judgment of the clinician, depending on the severity of pain and presence of other symptoms during the conservative treatment period.

the new practices, and we also expect to observe effects that are related to the particular intervention strategy of each MTF. For example, there should be a reduction in referrals to specialty care only for those MTFs that defined specialty referrals as a priority and actually undertook actions to reduce inappropriate referrals.

A Systems Approach to Implementation

A systems approach was applied in the AMEDD practice guideline implementation demonstrations, an approach that was amply supported by lessons from the demonstrations. The demonstrations highlighted that two main dimensions need to be addressed to ensure successful changes in practices by MTFs and other local facilities: (1) build local ownership or "buy-in" from the staff responsible for implementing the new practices, and (2) ensure that clinical and administrative systems are in place to facilitate staff adherence to the guideline.

Drawing on published literature and the experiences observed in the AMEDD demonstrations, we identified six critical success factors that strongly influence how successful an MTF will be in integrating new practices into its clinical and administrative processes (Chodoff and Crowley, 1995). In the evaluation, we assessed the performance of demonstration participants on these factors: (1) visible and consistent commitment by the MEDCOM leadership at all levels, (2) ongoing monitoring and reporting of implementation progress in carrying out an action plan, (3) implementation guidance to the MTFs by MEDCOM, (4) identification of an effective physician guideline champion at each MTF, (5) dedicated time and adequate resources for the guideline champions, and (6) rapid integration of new practices into a clinic's normal procedures.

The DoD/VA low back pain guideline was introduced in the Great Plains Region in November 1998 at the demonstration kickoff conference. The asthma guideline demonstration began in the Southeast Region in August 1999, and the diabetes guideline was introduced in the Western Region in December 1999. The guideline implementation process used in the demonstration consisted of (1) the practice guideline and metrics, (2) a guideline toolkit of materials to support the MTFs' implementation activities, (3) a kickoff planning conference at which demonstration MTF teams developed their implementation strategies and action plans, (4) MTF implementation activities following the kickoff conference to carry out the teams' action plans, (5) information exchange among the teams to share experiences and build on each other's successes, and (6) monitoring of implementation progress by both MEDCOM and the participating MTFs. Each demonstration was followed by Army-wide implementation of its guideline, beginning with the low back pain guideline in spring 2000.

The Demonstration Sites

Each demonstration was located in a different region to maximize the training and exposure of MTF personnel to the practice guidelines and implementation methods in preparation for systemwide implementation. The low back pain guideline demonstration was conducted with MTFs in the Army Great Plains Region. This region was selected for the first demonstration because it contains a large number and diversity of Army posts, MTFs, and populations served. A large number of all Army active duty personnel are stationed at Great Plains Region posts, and many military retirees and their dependents live within their catchment areas. Four MTFs in the Great Plains Region served as demonstration sites: William Beaumont Army Medical Center at Ft. Bliss, Darnall Army Community Hospital (ACH) at Ft. Hood, Evans ACH at Ft. Carson, and Reynolds ACH at Ft. Sill.

The four MTFs represented diverse patient populations, facility sizes, and service mixes. They also varied in other clinical and educational activities. At the time of the demonstration, two MTFs were sites for the DoD-Medicare Subvention Demonstration, in which the MTFs enrolled and provided services to Medicare-eligible DoD beneficiaries, and they also were chiropractic demonstration sites. These demonstrations changed their primary care service patterns. Chiropractic services historically had not been available in military facilities, so the other two MTFs did not have these services. The chiropractic demonstration was intended to generate information for use by DoD in deciding whether to provide chiropractic services in its health facilities.

THE RAND EVALUATION

The evaluation of the demonstration consisted of a process evaluation and an analysis of the effects of the guideline on service utilization. The specific methods and data used in the evaluation are described in Chapter Two and Appendix A.

In the process evaluation, the RAND team used a participant-observer approach to learn from and about the MTFs' experiences, to provide feedback, and to facilitate shared learning among the MTFs throughout the demonstration and evaluation process. The purposes of the process evaluation were to (1) document the actions and experiences of the participating MTFs and assess performance relative to each of the six critical success factors; (2) identify areas where AMEDD policies, systems, and processes can be strengthened; and (3) assess the degree to which MTFs can build on their experiences with the demonstration to implement additional DoD/VA guidelines.

In the process evaluation, we collected information from the participating MTFs through a series of site visits, monthly progress reports prepared by the MTFs, and questionnaires completed by individual participants. Three site visits were conducted at each demonstration site: an introductory visit before the kickoff conference, a post-implementation visit in June 1999 at three to four months after the MTFs began implementing the guideline, and a second post-implementation visit in February 2000 (at month nine or ten of implementation). During each post-implementation site visit, RAND staff interviewed the MTF's implementation team and others involved in changing practices in response to the new guideline. Summary reports of the results of the final round of site visits for the four participating MTFs are presented in Appendix B.

The purposes of the analysis of the effects of guideline implementation were to (1) document the extent to which intended actions were actually implemented by the MTFs; (2) monitor short-term effects on service delivery methods and activity, and where feasible, on client outcomes; and (3) develop metrics and measurement methods that can be adopted by the MTFs and MEDCOM for routine monitoring of progress.

An interrupted time series comparison-group design was used to assess the effects of the low back pain guideline demonstration. Quarterly administrative data on service utilization and medication prescriptions were collected for low back pain patients served by the demonstration and comparison (control) sites, which provided trend information both before and after introduction of the guideline in the Great Plains Region. The comparison group allowed us to control for temporal trends that might account for changes in the indicators. (See Chapter Two for the criteria and methods used to select comparison MTFs.) We selected indicators based on the hypotheses regarding effects of using conservative treatment for acute low back pain (listed above). The measures were appropriate choices for this demonstration because most of the participating MTFs focused their implementation actions on service delivery for acute low back pain (rather than chronic low back pain).

The patient population for this study was limited to active duty Army personnel who received care for acute low back pain at one of the demonstration or comparison sites during the time period of the study. This design was selected because we could not obtain complete pharmaceutical data for all patients using these MTFs. The pharmacy data constraint was important because use of pain medications is a major aspect of care for acute low back pain patients, and one-half of the indicators selected for the study are measures of pain medication use. Because acute low back pain is one of the major causes of lost duty days for active duty personnel, this study provides useful information even though it is limited to this population. We encourage expansion of the analysis to also include family members and retirees as other service utilization and pharmaceutical data become available.

KEY FINDINGS FROM THE DEMONSTRATION

This first demonstration to field test methods for implementation of clinical practice guidelines yielded rich insights even as the MTFs struggled to achieve lasting new practices. The performance of the demonstration and control MTFs on the six hypotheses for acute low back pain care (listed in the previous section of this summary) varied significantly at baseline (the six-month period before MTFs started working with the guideline). Introducing the guideline had few measurable effects related to those hypotheses. Despite these weak findings, the demonstration made a considerable contribution to improvements in methods for subsequent guideline demonstrations, and ultimately, for implementation of the low back pain guideline in all Army health facilities as of January 2000.

Two of the six critical success factors (see the previous section) emerged as the most important issues for the demonstration with respect to the limited success of the participating MTFs in improving low back pain care practices. Serious progress in practice improvement cannot happen without (1) having fully committed leadership at all levels and (2) establishing a credible monitoring and reporting system to provide accountability for desired improvements. The remaining four critical success factors contribute to the effectiveness and timeliness of actions, but they are not expected to support extensive progress in change if the leadership and monitoring are not in place.

Effects on Clinical Practices

At baseline, we found not only substantial variation across the demonstration and control MTFs on all six hypotheses, but also high levels of use of muscle relaxants, despite the guideline advice that muscle relaxants are not indicated. Muscle relaxants were prescribed for almost one-half of the acute low back pain patients. This baseline performance argues for proactive changes in practices for low back pain care to reduce variations and achieve the evidence-based practices specified in the practice guideline.

The implementation activities had only limited effects on care for low back pain patients during the first year the demonstration sites worked with the practice guideline. Also, the effects that were achieved were for service delivery rather than for prescribing of pain medications. The only overall effect for the demonstration was a decline in physical therapy referrals during the demonstration period. This effect was the result of large reductions in physical therapy referrals by two facilities that had established this goal as a priority in their implementation action plans.

The changes in service delivery that we observed typically could be identified with individual sites and were consistent with the site's implementation strategies. The strongest of these were the Site A strategy to use back classes to reduce use of physical therapy, which was observed in the data as declines in physical therapy referrals; and the Site D strategy to establish the physical medicine department as gatekeeper and reduce inappropriate specialty referrals, which was observed in the data as shifts of referrals to the physical medicine department from other specialties.

Performance on the Six Critical Factors

Research on practice guideline implementation has documented that a commitment to the implementation process, including use of multiple interventions, is required to achieve desired changes to clinical practices. This demonstration had mixed performance in the extent to which the six critical factors were realized, which affected the MTFs' progress in implementing practice improvements.

1. **Command leadership commitment at the MTF, regional, and corporate levels.** The AMEDD central and regional leadership expressed strong support for the demonstration, but initial verbal support was not followed by actions to provide resources to support the work or require active monitoring and reporting of the sites' performance in implementing new practices. Furthermore, the level of commitment by local MTF commanders varied, and changes in command further eroded support over time. This mixed response was understandable, given that this was the first demonstration in a new MEDCOM initiative and there were concerns regarding its effects on MTF workloads and costs. Many providers, including physicians in leadership roles, have instinctive negative reactions to practice guidelines as "cookbook medicine," which indeed we heard in our evaluation. Unfortunately, "wait and see" positions by command teams can become a self-fulfilling prophecy leading to failure of implementation efforts. We believe this lack of leadership commitment contributed to the limited results of the low back pain guideline demonstration.

2. **Monitoring of progress.** The demonstration did not perform well in the area of monitoring, in part because this was the first demonstration and it was put into the field very quickly, even as the DoD/VA practice guideline was still being completed. The guideline expert panel did not select the key metrics for systemwide monitoring until well into the demonstration period. Further, MEDCOM did not have the resources to establish a monitoring system at the corpo-

rate level. Without structured guidance from the corporate level, the sites varied widely in their approach to monitoring, and most did not routinely measure their progress in introducing new practices or effects on service delivery patterns. Not having such data is important because, in the absence of objective evidence, providers and clinic staff tend to believe that they are performing well and either do not have to make changes or that changes they made were successful. These beliefs are often overly optimistic.

3. **Guidance and support to the MTFs by MEDCOM.** MEDCOM made a solid commitment to providing the MTFs with policy guidance and technical support to enhance their ability to implement best practices for low back pain treatment. Such support can also encourage consistent practices across the Army facilities. The nature of this support evolved during the demonstration, ultimately including preparation of a toolkit of support materials, hands-on technical support through site visits, and coordination of information exchange among the MTFs. MEDCOM staff limitations led to some delays in preparing the low back pain toolkit materials, especially at the start of the demonstration. We believe this committed support by MEDCOM has been a powerful foundation for the practice improvements achieved in the guideline demonstrations, as MEDCOM learned from each field test and applied those lessons to subsequent demonstrations.

4. **Guideline champions who are opinion leaders.** From the start, MEDCOM identified Army-wide guideline champions who were respected leaders with a commitment to using the guideline to improve the quality of care. The participating MTFs also identified well-respected physicians to serve as guideline champions, and most of these physicians showed a commitment to leading the implementation activities for their facilities. Some of the initial champions were replaced in the course of the demonstration because of rotations and deployments. This demonstration highlighted that it sometimes will be difficult to find a champion who both has enthusiasm for the guideline and is a respected opinion leader, and at times, facilities will have to make trade-offs between these factors.

5. **Resource support for champions.** All of the MTF commanders designated champions to lead the implementation of the guideline, but few of the champions received tangible support for their activi-

ties (other than attendance at the kickoff conference). Most of them had to perform the implementation work in addition to their regular workload. In most of the MTFs, a facilitator designated by the MTF commander provided staff support to the champion, and for some facilitators, this role was an integral part of their regular job. The need to do "double duty" means that champions are able to make only a time-limited commitment to such an initiative, after which they either "burn out" or must turn their attention to other priorities. Thus it is important to integrate new practices into ongoing procedures as quickly and effectively as possible, within the available time of the champion.

6. **Institutionalization of new practices.** Staff turnover or shifts in policies at the command level can destabilize efforts to introduce and sustain new practices. Three of the participating MTFs made early progress in achieving practices consistent with the low back pain guideline. The fourth MTF viewed low back pain as a low priority and planned few practice changes. Two of the active sites lost momentum over time, one because of heavy workload demands related to deployments, and the other because of changing priorities associated with changes in command. Only one site achieved practice changes that are likely to remain in place. These changes have a good chance of surviving because they addressed an issue that was important to providers and MTF leadership. We note, however, that even successful practice changes may be vulnerable to later policy shifts with subsequent changes in MTF leadership, which occur about every three years.

LESSONS FROM THE CORPORATE PERSPECTIVE

A primary goal of the low back pain guideline demonstration, as well as of the subsequent demonstrations for the asthma and diabetes guidelines, was to test and refine a corporate system for implementing evidence-based best practices as specified in the guidelines. Thus, our evaluation was interested in the experiences of the participating MTFs as they introduced new practices as well as in the effects of those practices, to the extent they were effectively put into place, on clinical practices for low back pain.

Guided by the experiences of the low back pain, asthma, and diabetes demonstrations, an effective corporate implementation strategy emerged over time for practice guideline implementation across the Army Medical Department. The field experience bore out the value of using a systems approach, in this case including both corporate and local roles. Continuous quality improvement techniques served well in planning and carrying out the implementation steps, showing the value of using a series of incremental steps, each of which builds upon previous steps to achieve continual improvements in health care processes and outcomes over time.

Given the weak effects on clinical practices found for the low back pain guideline, however, further work is needed to focus the attention of the leadership and strengthen actions to achieve the practices supported by scientific evidence. The following specific action items emerged from the low back pain demonstration that are within MEDCOM's authority and responsibility:

- Maintain the proactive role of MEDCOM in managing a coordinated guideline implementation program across the system, including the responsiveness it has shown to MTFs as they have pursued local implementation activities. MEDCOM has eased the workload for MTFs by providing tools and technical guidance, thus enhancing the potential to achieve practice improvements.
- To support the establishment of a system-level monitoring process to track MTF progress in improving clinical practices, develop the data and analytic capability to perform measurements and report results to the MTFs. The analytic function should be equipped to provide training and support to MTFs for their local monitoring processes.
- When introducing a new practice guideline for MTF implementation, provide clear guidance and instructions so the MTFs know what is expected of them and where they have the flexibility to act locally. Set objectives and define which aspects are mandated and which are left to MTF discretion. Maintain a balance between flexibility for local MTF approaches and sufficient policy direction to be sure that AMEDD is moving toward greater consistency in practices.

- Provide resources to support implementation activities at levels commensurate with the expected workload and results, including resources for both MEDCOM and the MTFs.
- Reevaluate the MEDCOM policy on the use of standard forms in the management of care for conditions addressed by the practice guidelines. Although the low back pain documentation form was shown to improve provider efficiency, it became a point of contention that often distracted from the real task at hand. The number of new forms will multiply as more guidelines are introduced, which could be detrimental for the program if not presented appropriately.
- Develop contractual mechanisms to ensure that contract providers participate in implementing improved practices and to ensure that MEDCOM is able to monitor the performance of these providers using the same metrics applied to the MTFs. Contract providers resisted participation for the low back pain guideline, and they were not actively involved in other demonstrations. These attitudes are due in part to financial incentives created by their contracts, where they are paid based on the number of visits they complete, and time spent on any other activities is unpaid time.
- Provide proactive MEDCOM leadership for ensuring information exchange among MTFs. Individual MTFs are not likely to volunteer for the extra work involved in taking the lead in communicating with others without incentives and support from above.
- Provide guidance and training to the MTFs on how to perform effective patient education as part of the treatment of conditions covered by practice guidelines, including techniques for encouraging patients to assume greater responsibility for self-care.
- Pay attention to the details of the many issues the MTFs raise as they work with a guideline. Examples of issues that occurred in the low back pain demonstration (as well as later in the asthma and diabetes guideline demonstrations) include how to handle patients presenting with multiple concerns or diagnoses, placement of documentation forms in the medical chart, procedures for use of diagnostic codes for visits, and reading levels for patient education materials.

- Managing care according to the DoD/VA practice guidelines represents a proactive primary care management approach for patients with specific health conditions. Thus, consider replacing traditional utilization review functions with this more proactive approach to achieve appropriate and consistent practices.

LESSONS FOR THE TREATMENT FACILITIES

As we observed the experiences of the participating MTFs during the demonstration, several items surfaced that MTFs are likely to face regularly in implementation efforts:

- Momentum (or lack of it) will strongly influence progress in achieving new practices. Therefore, teams should strive to capitalize on the momentum generated by the start-up activities when the team is defining problems and preparing its action plan. Two essential elements are to quickly go into the field to test new ideas, and to frequently communicate what is being learned with those not on the team.
- Command leadership commitment is necessary for changing clinical practices, but alone it is not a sufficient ingredient. Leadership must hold the teams accountable for following through on implementation actions, monitoring progress, and achieving their goals.
- The best chance of establishing lasting new clinic procedures requires the sincere involvement by all clinic staff. It is worth taking the time required to educate all potential participants about the goals and contents of a guideline and to build their understanding and acceptance of the best practices being introduced.
- Action plans need to evolve and change over time. Even the best designed and executed action plan is unlikely to change the practices of all patients and providers. Ongoing monitoring will suggest new areas that need to be addressed, and continuing interventions will be needed to sustain and spread changes needed for full compliance with practice standards by all those involved.
- Among the first actions that should be taken in implementing new practices are to define the metrics for monitoring and to work with the appropriate offices to get the necessary data. Ide-

ally, the implementation team should establish the capability to provide monitoring feedback to its MTF clinics within a month or two after beginning implementation of new clinical practices.

- Personnel rotations are an ongoing part of military life, and they should not be an excuse for lack of progress on implementing improved practices. As each MTF defines its action plan and schedule, it should anticipate and plan for military rotations, including effects on the clinic staff and on the members of the implementation team itself. Any surprise personnel movements that affect staffing can be accommodated by action plan updates and revisions.

ACKNOWLEDGMENTS

An extraordinary amount of dedication and hard work by numerous individuals contributed to the performance of the AMEDD demonstration for implementing the DoD/VA low back pain guideline in the Great Plains Region. In particular, we wish to acknowledge the efforts of the guideline champions, facilitators, and action team members at the Army treatment facilities—William Beaumont AMC, Darnall ACH, Evans ACH, and Reynolds ACH—participating in the demonstration. Because this was the first demonstration, these individuals were faced with delays and other challenges during the early months, as MEDCOM, RAND, and the MTFs themselves experienced a steep learning curve—the proverbial "learning by doing." These teams persisted in their implementation efforts, achieving observable progress in changing clinical practices and offering invaluable feedback on how to make the process stronger and more efficient.

We also acknowledge the commitment of the leadership team members at MEDCOM who have guided this project and have participated as active partners in both the development and evaluation work on the low back pain demonstration. LTC Kathryn Dolter, who has primary responsibility for the MEDCOM guideline implementation program, has shown unflagging commitment to learning from our demonstrations and making this important program come to life. Her willingness to lead and to listen to those in the field have been critical factors in the progress made to date. The personnel in the Patient Administration Systems and Biostatistical Activity (PASBA) also made a major contribution to the evaluation by generating the administrative data for the analysis of the effects of guideline implementation. Their careful data extraction and programming efforts ensured the needed data integrity. Without the policy and financial support of the Center for Healthcare Education and Studies, headed by COL Harrison Hassell, this project would not have been possible.

Finally, we offer our thanks to our RAND colleagues Paul Shekelle and Marge Pearson for their thoughtful review of an earlier draft of this final report. Their suggestions for revisions helped to make it a stronger document. Any errors of fact or interpretation are, of course, the responsibility of the authors and not of any of those who provided feedback on our efforts.

ACRONYMS AND ABBREVIATIONS

ACH	Army community hospital
ADS	Ambulatory Data System
AMC	Army medical center
AMEDD	Army Medical Department
CBC	complete blood count
CEIS	Corporate Executive Information System
CHCS	the MTFs' clinical information system
CHES	Center for Health Education and Studies
CHPPM	Center for Health Promotion and Preventive Medicine
CIW	Clinical Integrated Workplace
CME	continuing medical education
CTMC	Consolidated Troop Medical Clinic
DoD	Department of Defense
ER	emergency room
ESR	erythrocyte sedimentation rate
FY	fiscal year
KMN	Knowledge Management Network
MEB	Medical Evaluation Board

MEDCOM	United States Army Medical Command
MEPRS	Medical Expense and Performance Report System for Fixed Military Medical and Dental Treatment Facilities
MTF	military/medical treatment facility
NSAID	nonsteroidal anti-inflammatory drug
PA	physician assistant
PASBA	Patient Administration Systems and Biostatistical Activity
PEC	PharmacoEconomic Center
PT	physical therapy
QI	quality improvement
QM	quality management
SADR	Standard Ambulatory Data Record
SIDPERS	Standard Installation/Division Personnel System
TMC	troop medical clinic
UM	utilization management
USPD	Uniformed Services Prescription Database
VA	Veterans Affairs, Department of

Chapter One

INTRODUCTION

The Army Medical Department (AMEDD) is committed to establishing a structure and process to support its military/medical treatment facilities (MTFs) in implementing evidence-based practice guidelines to achieve best practices that reduce variation and enhance quality of medical care. AMEDD contracted with the RAND Corporation to work as a partner in the development and testing of guideline implementation methods for ultimate application in an Army-wide guideline program.

Taking the approach of testing new methods on a small scale, the AMEDD/RAND project fielded three sequential demonstrations over a two-year period, in each of which participating MTFs implemented a different clinical practice guideline. All of the demonstrations worked with practice guidelines that were established collaboratively by the Departments of Veterans Affairs (VA) and Defense (DoD). In the first demonstration, four MTFs in the Great Plains Region implemented the practice guideline for low back pain. The asthma guideline was implemented by four MTFs in the Southeast Region, and the diabetes guideline was implemented by two MTFs in the Western Region.

RAND performed evaluations for each demonstration that included a process evaluation and an analysis of effects on service delivery. Specific components of this work included the following:

- *Process evaluation* documented the implementation activities of participating MTFs, described their successes in changing clinical practices, identified successes and challenges reported by the sites, and obtained their feedback regarding U.S. Army Medical Command (MEDCOM) support.

- *Analysis of effects* estimated the extent to which the sites' implementation activities affected specific measures of service delivery for low back pain, with comparisons to a control group of MTFs that did not implement the guideline.
- *Benchmarking* described variations in practices across MTFs for the measures used in the analysis of effects to help identify priorities for future interventions and for comparing individual facilities to benchmarks for target levels of performance.
- *Methods development* documented the measurement methods developed and related data requirements to provide a basis for future systemwide monitoring of progress in achieving best practices for each condition addressed by a guideline.

This report presents the results from our evaluation of the implementation of the low back pain guideline in the Great Plains Region demonstration. These findings build on and extend the results of our process evaluation of the first three months of activity for the low back pain demonstration.[1] The remainder of this chapter summarizes the process DoD and the VA used to establish practice guidelines and MEDCOM's approach to implementing the guidelines in the Army environment. Chapter Two describes the methods and data used for the evaluation. Chapter Three reports the benchmarking of baseline performance of the nine MTFs in the study on each of the six measures (see Table 3.1) of low back pain services used to assess the effects of the guideline on clinical practices. Results of the process evaluation are reported in Chapters Four and Five, and results of the evaluation of guideline effects are presented in Chapter Six. Finally, in Chapter Seven we synthesize the results of the full evaluation and identify lessons learned, issues to be addressed, and implications for systemwide guideline implementation strategies.

---

[1]Unpublished RAND research by Donna O. Farley, Georges Vernez, Elaine S. Quiter, and Shan Cretin.

THE DoD/VA GUIDELINE ADAPTATION PROCESS

DoD and the VA initiated a collaborative project in early 1998 to establish a single standard of care in the military and VA health systems. This project is led by a working group consisting of two representatives from each of the three military services and the VA. The goals of this project are (1) adaptation of existing clinical practice guidelines for selected conditions, (2) selection of two to four indicators for each guideline to benchmark and monitor implementation progress, and (3) integration of DoD/VA prevention, pharmaceutical, and clinical informatics efforts.

The DoD/VA working group designated an expert panel for each practice guideline, consisting of representatives from the three military services and the VA, with a mix of clinical backgrounds relevant to the health condition of interest. The expert panel reviewed existing national guidelines for that condition, examined and updated the scientific evidence supporting the guidelines, and established an adaptation of one or more of the guidelines for use in the military and veteran health systems. Each panel was also asked to develop recommendations to the DoD/VA guideline working group for the metrics to be used by the military services and the VA to monitor progress in guideline implementation.

With this approach to guideline development, DoD and the VA have made a commitment to use of evidence-based practices in their health care facilities. Each practice guideline is a statement of best practices for the management and treatment of the health condition it addresses. The recommendations for practices in each component of care take into account the strength of relevant scientific evidence, which is documented in the practice guideline report. The guidelines support substantial clinical discretion on the part of the provider, while identifying areas where specific practices are either strongly advised or not advised. In areas where scientific evidence is weak, the guideline notes that recommendations are based on the collective clinical judgment of the expert panel.

OVERVIEW OF THE PRACTICE GUIDELINE FOR LOW BACK PAIN

The principal emphasis of the DoD/VA practice guideline for primary care management of low back pain is on acute low back pain, which is defined as low back pain occurring during the first six weeks after the initial onset of pain (VHA/DoD, 1999). Five key guideline elements were identified by the expert panel responsible for the low back pain guideline, which are presented in Table 1.1. As described in key element 2, the guideline recommends use of conservative treatment (minimal clinical intervention) for acute low back pain patients to allow recovery to take place naturally, which occurs in 80–90 percent of these patients. Patients should be educated on self-care management techniques, including reduction in activity and light exercises to help ease the pain. Imaging studies or laboratory tests are not recommended initially except for cases with symptoms indicating the presence of a more serious condition. Pain medications may be used to ease patients' discomfort, but these should not include muscle relaxants. Patients with more intense, continuing pain may be referred to physical therapy or manipulation to assist the healing process.

EXPECTED EFFECTS ON HEALTH CARE PRACTICES

The emphasis of the low back pain guideline on conservative treatment for patients with acute low back pain (the first six weeks following the initial low back pain visit) should be the primary driver of any changes in clinical practices that might be observed as the MTFs implemented the guideline. For chronic low back pain patients (those who still have pain after six weeks), care should become more proactive, including additional diagnostic tests and consultation and referral to specialists as appropriate.

To the extent that facilities have been treating acute low back pain patients more aggressively than the guideline recommends, we would expect to see reductions in the use of manipulation (by physical therapy or chiropractic), in the frequency of primary care visits, in specialty referrals, in imaging studies, in laboratory tests, and in prescriptions for pain medications during the first six weeks of care. For

Table 1.1

Key Elements of the DoD/VA Practice Guideline for Low Back Pain

Key Element	Description
1. Evaluation for Serious Health Problems	
Accurate and timely identification should be made of clinical conditions for which low back pain is a symptom, which should be managed appropriately with consultation or referred for specialty care.	When examining the patient, (a) the primary care practitioner should look for red flags that indicate the presence of one of these conditions. (b) If red flags are found, patients who are emergent or urgent cases should be identified for immediate consultation or referral. (c) For nonemergent cases with red flags, appropriate diagnostic tests should be ordered to assess whether the patient has a condition that requires referral.
2. Symptom Control for Acute Low Back Pain Patients	
For low back pain patients who do not have another identifiable health problem, symptom control should be the first line treatment (conservative treatment).	Depending on the patient, (a) treatment may include appropriate use of activity modification, bed rest, conservative medication, progressive range of motion and exercise, manipulative treatment, and education. (b) Such treatment should be used for 4–6 weeks before performing additional evaluation or diagnostic tests, unless the patient gets worse. (c) Contact with the patient should be maintained to monitor progress and adjust treatment as indicated.
3. Evaluation of Patients Whose Condition Gets Worse	
Low back pain patients whose condition gets worse during the time their symptoms are treated should be identified and reevaluated quickly, with consultation or referral as appropriate.	(a) During periodic contact with the patient, questions should be asked to identify any deterioration in the patient's condition, including new neurological symptoms, increase in pain, new radiation of pain, or other symptoms. (b) When such problems are found, the patient should be reevaluated for other emergent or nonemergent health problems, with consults or referral when indicated.
4. Evaluation of Patients Who Do Not Improve	
Patients whose low back pain does not improve after 4–6 weeks should be further evaluated for evidence of an underlying medical condition or psychosocial problems.	These patients are considered to have chronic low back pain or sciatica. (a) A history and physical examination should be performed to rule out other serious problems, and (b) psychosocial distress and risk factors should be explored using self-report questionnaires.

Table 1.1—continued

Key Element	Description
5. Management of Chronic Low Back Pain or Sciatica	
Different diagnostic tests and management strategies should be used for patients with chronic low back pain and patients with chronic sciatica.	(a) A patient with pain radiating past the knee should be classified as having chronic sciatica, with diagnostic tests performed to inform decisions regarding surgical consult or referral. (b) A patient with no radiating pain should be classified as having chronic low back pain, with diagnostic tests performed to inform decisions regarding medical management, including consultation or referral to medical specialists. (c) Active duty personnel with chronic low back pain or sciatica that has not improved in 4 to 6 months should be assessed for referral to the Medical Evaluation Board for possible reclassification or discharge from service.

SOURCE: AMEDD, 1999.

chronic low back pain patients, changes might occur in use of specialty care and diagnostic tests. The changes for chronic patients might include increases over previous practices because the guideline offers direction to primary care providers that could encourage them to treat these patients more proactively than they had previously.

Given the guideline emphasis on conservative treatment for acute low back pain patients, our analyses focused on patterns of service delivery and pain medication prescriptions during the conservative treatment period. We tested the hypotheses that increased use of conservative treatment (i.e., less aggressive clinical intervention) for acute low back pain patients will lead to a decrease in the following clinical practices during the first six weeks of care:[2]

1. percentage of patients referred to physical therapy or manipulation
2. number of follow-up visits per low back pain patient

---

[2]These measures do not include any of the DoD/VA metrics because the DoD/VA metrics could not be measured with readily available administrative data and do not address early effects of use of the guideline.

3. percentage of acute low back pain patients referred to specialty care
4. percentage of acute low back pain patients prescribed muscle relaxants
5. percentage of acute low back pain patients prescribed narcotics
6. percentage of nonsteroidal anti-inflammatory drugs (NSAIDs) prescribed that are high cost.

Three other hypotheses addressing possible practice changes for acute low back pain patients were defined, but they could not be analyzed because the needed data were not available. The MTFs reported inpatient and outpatient encounters routinely in the DoD central health database, but there was no central reporting of ancillary service data. These hypotheses stated that use of conservative treatment for acute low back pain patients would be associated with reduction in

- ordering of X rays and other diagnostic imaging
- complete blood count and erythrocyte sedimentation rate testing of patients with no red-flag conditions
- lost or restricted duty days.

We developed additional hypotheses regarding guideline effects for chronic low back pain and incidence of new episodes of care, which also could be tracked in ongoing monitoring of low back pain care. Hypotheses regarding chronic low back pain state that more proactive management of patients with chronic low back pain would be associated with

- increased ordering of X ray and other diagnostic imaging after six weeks of primary care treatment
- increased referrals to specialists after six weeks of treatment
- more prompt referrals to specialists following X ray or other diagnostic imaging that occurs more than six weeks after the initial low back pain visit (for those referred)
- decrease in referrals of chronic low back pain or sciatica patients to the Medical Evaluation Board because more effective man-

agement of their low back pain would enable more of them to recover more fully and return to active duty.

As an MTF adjusted its practices to be consistent with the low back pain guideline, more aggressive patient education and management practices would be undertaken that should influence patients to use more prevention and self-care, which in turn should affect incidence of new episodes of care. Therefore, we also hypothesized that the new practices would lead to (1) a decrease in the incidence of new low back pain visits among active duty personnel and (2) a decrease in entry of low back pain patients through the emergency room and specialists.

A SYSTEMS APPROACH TO IMPLEMENTATION

Most studies that have evaluated the effects of guideline implementation on health care practices have been fairly narrow studies of individual interventions to change provider behavior (e.g., education, audit and feedback, and reminders), primarily due to researchers' efforts to design studies with effective controls. Results across studies are quite variable, explained partly by differences in subject matter of the guideline, provider attitudes, and organizational characteristics (Grilli and Lomas, 1994; Chodoff and Crowley, 1995; Eastwood and Sheldon, 1996). The results are often disappointing, as in the finding that nearly one-third of the time primary care providers fail to follow even noncontroversial and evidence-based guideline recommendations (Grol et al., 1998). Active methods, such as concurrent reminders and academic detailing, are more consistently effective than passive dissemination of guidelines or feedback. Combining two or more approaches seems more likely to succeed than relying on a single intervention (Bero et al., 1998).

Influenced by a systems approach and quality improvement, health care managers favor multifaceted changes in systems, rather than single interventions, as the best hope for changing patient care practices (Senge, 1990; Shortell, Bennett, and Byck, 1998). The Chronic Care Model, for example, suggests that care of the chronically ill requires major changes in the organization and delivery of care, in information systems, in doctor-patient relationships, in patient self-management, and even in relationships between the health system and community resources (Wagner, Austin, and Von Korff, 1996; Von Korff et al., 1997). A premise of this and other integrated models is that testing the effects of individual components will yield misleading null results, since dramatic changes in outcome *only* occur when all components of the model are in place. Distinguishing, as Hargraves et al. (1996) do, between provider-controlled and system-dependent guideline criteria is difficult. System changes (such as computerized order entry linked to decision support) can clearly change the degree of compliance with practitioner-controlled criteria, such as choice of antibiotic (Evans et al., 1998).

Basic Implementation Strategy

A systems approach was applied in the AMEDD practice guideline demonstrations—an approach that was amply supported by lessons from the demonstrations that documented the importance of addressing multiple factors that influence clinical practices. The experiences of the MTFs participating in the low back pain demonstration highlighted the need for a coherent strategy for achieving lasting change. Two main dimensions need to be addressed to ensure successful changes in practices by MTFs and other local facilities: (1) build local ownership or "buy-in" from the staff responsible for implementing the new practices and (2) ensure that clinical and administrative systems are in place to facilitate staff adherence to the guideline.

We show graphically in Figure 1.1 how staff buy-in and system changes interact to produce different implementation results. Having *both* local ownership and system support produces the optimal result, leading to likely implementation success. System support without local ownership produces providers who are resistant to implementation, despite having clinic procedures and systems equipped to support the process. Provider ownership without system support produces providers who wish to change practices but are frustrated at their inability to overcome barriers in the MTF systems that hamper their ability to do so. Finally, with *neither* local ownership nor system support, implementation will fail.

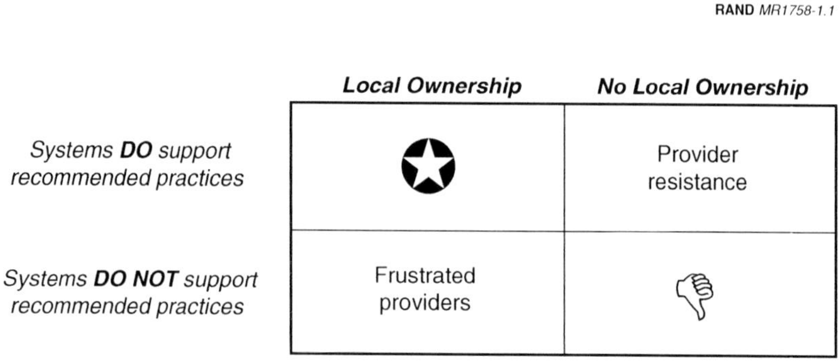

Figure 1.1—Matrix of Implementation Outcomes

Six Critical Success Factors

Drawing upon published literature, we identified six critical success factors that influence how successful a health care organization will be in integrating lasting change into its clinical and administrative processes. Lessons from the AMEDD demonstrations provided empirical support for the importance of these factors:

1. Visible and consistent commitment by command leadership at the MTF, regional, and corporate levels. Without it, effective practice changes are not likely to occur.

2. Ongoing monitoring of progress in carrying out an implementation action plan, to be performed by both the MTFs and MEDCOM, with regular feedback to the MTFs on the effects of their actions on desired outcomes.

3. Provision of implementation guidance and support to the MTFs by MEDCOM, including toolkits of support materials and ready access to staff support and other resources. Such support encourages MTFs to make needed practice changes to move toward consistency in practices across the Army facilities.

4. Identification of a physician at each MTF, who is a respected local opinion leader, to serve as guideline champion and lead the MTF's implementation activities.

5. Provision of adequate dedicated time and other resource support for the guideline champions to enable them to perform their tasks effectively. Such support will also reinforce the signals that guideline implementation is a priority for the MTF command.
6. Institutionalization of new practices as part of a clinic's normal (routine) procedures within a finite time period (typically six months or less). This requires successful design and execution of an action plan to change practices, including both educational and systems change interventions.

THE AMEDD/RAND GUIDELINE IMPLEMENTATION PROJECT

The goal of the AMEDD/RAND project was to establish a system for implementing selected practice guidelines throughout the Army Medical Department, including monitoring the effects of those guidelines on clinical care and outcomes. Three sequential demonstrations were conducted that allowed AMEDD, RAND, and the participating MTFs to test and refine guideline implementation methods. As shown in Figure 1.2, each demonstration served as a "continuous quality improvement" cycle through which a regional test preceded systemwide implementation of a practice guideline. As the demonstrations progressed, RAND performed process evaluations to learn from the experiences of participating MTFs, and the cumulative results of the evaluations guided preparation for each subsequent demonstration. At the same time, MEDCOM began preparations to implement the guideline in all MTFs across the Army health system.

The DoD/VA low back pain guideline was introduced in the Great Plains Region in November 1998 at the demonstration kickoff conference. The asthma guideline demonstration began in the Southeast Region in August 1999, and the diabetes guideline was introduced in the Western Region in December 1999. Army-wide implementation of the low back pain guideline began in spring 2000. The guideline implementation process shown in Figure 1.3 was the systems approach applied in the demonstrations, which consisted of the following components:

RAND MR1758-1.2

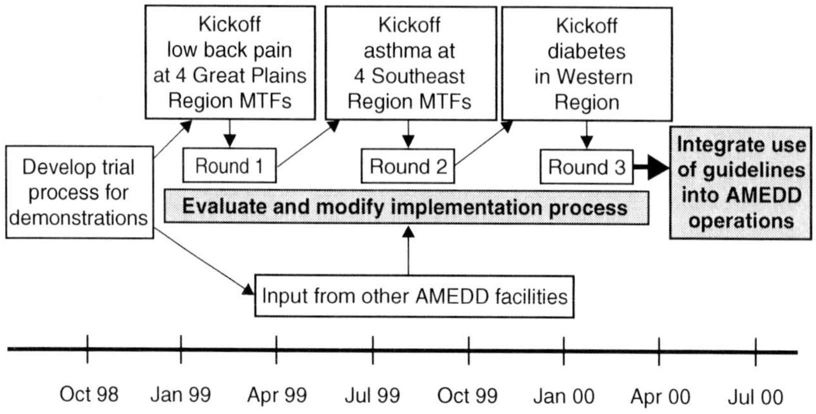

Figure 1.2—Diagram of the Demonstration Project

RAND MR1758-1.3

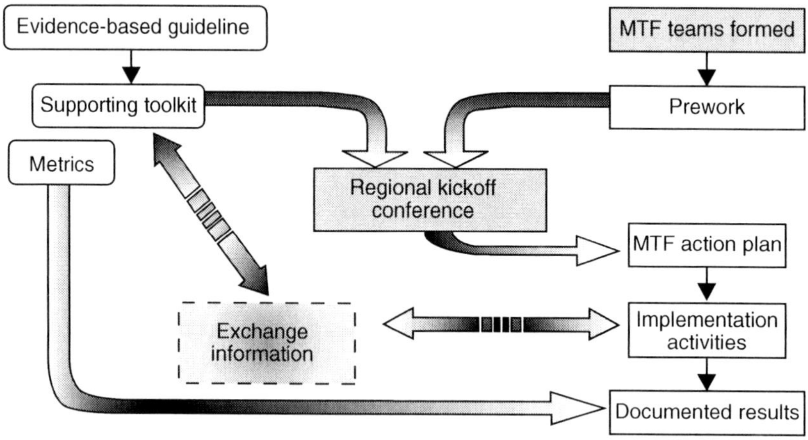

Figure 1.3—Guideline Implementation Process

- ***Practice guideline and metrics.*** The official DoD/VA practice guideline materials were provided to the MTFs, including a summary list of the key elements of the guideline and metrics identified by the guideline expert panel for monitoring progress.
- ***Guideline toolkit.*** MEDCOM and the Center for Health Promotion and Preventive Medicine (CHPPM) collaborated in the development of a toolkit of materials to support the MTFs' guideline implementation activities (e.g., documentation forms, provider training videos, patient education materials, and reminder cards).
- ***Kickoff planning conference.*** Multidisciplinary teams from the demonstration MTFs participated in a two-day meeting to develop their guideline implementation strategies and action plans.
- ***MTF implementation activities.*** Following the kickoff conference, the MTF teams carried out their action plans. They prepared monthly reports that summarized their recent activities, successes, challenges, and assistance needed to support their work.
- ***Information exchange.*** Teams were encouraged to share their experiences and build on each other's successes.
- ***Monitoring of progress.*** Monitoring of implementation progress was performed by both MEDCOM and the participating MTFs, using metrics that were developed either in the DoD/VA guideline process or by the MTFs. The MTFs were encouraged to establish measures for their key action strategies so they can assess their progress in making the clinical process changes they intended.

THE DEMONSTRATION SITES

The Great Plains Region was selected for the low back pain guideline demonstration because of the size and diversity of the posts located in the region and the populations they serve. These posts provide basic and/or advanced training for active duty personnel, including field artillery, air defense artillery, and armored cavalry. A large number of the Army active duty personnel are stationed at Great Plains Region posts, and many military retirees and their dependents live within their catchment areas. Therefore, the Great Plains Region medical treatment facilities are serving patients ranging from soldiers in basic training to Medicare-eligible retirees and dependents.

As shown in Table 1.2, the four MTFs in the Great Plains Region that served as demonstration sites for implementation of the low back pain guideline represent diverse patient populations, facility sizes, and service mixes. As Army community hospitals (ACH), Evans, Darnall, and Reynolds provide mainly primary care services with some specialty care. William Beaumont Army Medical Center (AMC) had a focus on specialty care services prior to 1996 but, during the time of the demonstration, was shifting to a mix of primary care and specialty care. The patient populations served by Darnall ACH and Reynolds ACH are primarily active duty personnel and dependents, whereas William Beaumont AMC serves a relatively large retiree population, as does Evans ACH to a lesser extent. The ratios of retirees to active duty personnel range from a low of 0.96 at Darnall ACH to a high of 2.87 at William Beaumont AMC.

The four MTFs also varied in other clinical and educational activities. Darnall ACH and William Beaumont AMC had extensive medical ed-

Table 1.2

Profiles of the Military Treatment Facilities Participating in the Low Back Pain Guideline Demonstration

	Evans ACH Ft. Carson, CO	Darnall ACH Ft. Hood, TX	Reynolds ACH Ft. Sill, OK	Beaumont AMC Ft. Bliss, TX
Number of beneficiaries				
Active duty	15,543	41,396	16,508	11,425
Active duty dependents	26,322	52,344	17,751	18,748
Retirees, dependents, and survivors	26,794	39,680	18,601	32,836
All beneficiaries	69,205	134,308	53,588	64,015
Ratio of retiree/active duty	1.72	0.96	1.13	2.87
Inpatient dispositions*	1,470	2,731	1,914	2,234
Same day surgeries*	631	1,423	1,180	2,065
Outpatient visits*	166,418	256,500	158,499	118,188

NOTE: All data are from Corporate Executive Information System (CEIS), 1999. Asterisked items are for the period October 1998–March 1999. All other data are from fiscal year 1998.

ucation training. Evans ACH and William Beaumont AMC had wellness centers. Evans ACH and Reynolds ACH were sites for the DoD-Medicare Subvention Demonstration, in which the MTFs enrolled and provided services to Medicare-eligible DoD beneficiaries. These two MTFs were also chiropractic demonstration sites, which changed their primary care service patterns. Chiropractic services historically had not been available in military facilities, so the other two MTFs did not have these services. The chiropractic demonstration was intended to generate information for use by DoD in deciding whether to provide chiropractic services in its health facilities. Sites varied widely in their previous experience with clinical practice guidelines or pathways. Access to and sophistication of computer support also varied considerably.

THE RAND EVALUATION

The evaluation of the demonstration by RAND consisted of two components: a process evaluation and an analysis of the effects of the guideline on clinical practices. The purposes and approaches of these evaluation components are presented here; the methods and data used are described in Chapter Two and Appendix A.

The Process Evaluation

To learn from the experience of the MTFs participating in the demonstration, the RAND team used a participant-observer approach to exchange information and facilitate shared learning with the MTFs throughout the demonstration and evaluation process. The purposes of the process evaluation were to

- document the actions and experiences of the Army MTFs participating in the demonstration for practice guideline implementation and assess performance relative to each of the six critical success factors
- identify areas where the policies, systems, and processes established by AMEDD for guideline implementation can be strengthened

- assess the degree to which demonstration sites are able to build on their experiences with the demonstration guideline to implement additional DoD/VA guidelines.

To understand the full dynamics of a process as complex as practice guideline implementation, we gathered information on the interactions of the many aspects of the system in which the guidelines were being implemented and the roles of a variety of stakeholders. These groups included the implementation team, treatment program leadership, middle management, the clinical and administrative staff working with program residents, and the clients themselves. To capture changes in structures and processes as guideline implementation moved forward, information was collected at baseline and at two follow-up points in time during site visits to capture (1) early lessons from the implementation activities and (2) information on successes and challenges in implementing desired new practices.

Analysis of Guideline Effects

The purposes of the analysis of the effects of guideline implementation were to

- document the changes in clinical process and service activity in a program that is implementing a practice guideline
- document changes in clinical practices that are attributable to the process changes that have occurred
- develop metrics and measurement methods that can be adopted by the participating programs for routine monitoring of their continued progress on an ongoing basis.

The first two purposes were the essence of the evaluation activities for the time period of the demonstration. However, the importance of the third purpose cannot be overstated. A viable monitoring process, including well-chosen, relevant measures, is essential for an MTF to be able to retain the gains it achieves by modifying practices as recommended by the guideline. This feedback loop continues to provide MTF staff with program quality information, and it maintains the visibility of the measures being reported as priorities for quality performance.

Chapter Two

METHODS AND DATA

The RAND evaluation for the low back pain guideline demonstration gathered information about both the processes of implementing the practice guideline at participating MTFs and the effects of these implementation activities on delivery of care for low back pain patients. In this chapter, we summarize the methods and data for these two evaluation components. Additional details are provided in Appendix A.

Implementation of a clinical practice guideline is one type of quality improvement intervention. An evaluation of any quality improvement intervention should recognize the incremental nature of these processes, which require time to achieve lasting practice improvements. A comprehensive evaluation of guideline implementation, therefore, would encompass the following three phases of emphasis:

1. **Introducing new practices.** Initial evaluation emphasis is on documenting the extent to which effective action plans are developed and the intended actions are actually implemented. Process evaluation methods are used here, and feedback to participants is provided early in the process and is designed to help them strengthen their interventions.

2. **Achieving intended changes in practices.** Subsequent emphasis is on monitoring short-term effects of the quality improvement interventions on service delivery methods and activity, applying a combination of process and impact (outcome) evaluation methods. The impact evaluation works with quantifiable measures that are relevant to the desired changes in either clinical processes or proximal outcomes.

3. **Improving patient outcomes.** Final emphasis takes a longer-term perspective, assessing the effects of program changes on client outcomes. This evaluation step uses outcome evaluation methods exclusively. Many of the measures developed to assess effects in the second and third evaluation phases can be used by the programs for ongoing monitoring.

The RAND evaluation for the low back pain guideline demonstration encompasses the first two evaluation phases. Lessons were drawn from the implementation process itself to strengthen future guideline implementation activities (introducing new practices), and data were analyzed to assess the early effects of the low back pain guideline on health care processes (achieving intended changes in practices).

PROCESS EVALUATION METHODS

In the process evaluation for the low back pain guideline demonstration, we collected information from the participating MTFs through a series of site visits, monthly progress reports prepared by participating MTFs, and questionnaires completed by individual participants. Additional details on these methods are presented in Appendix A.

Three visits were conducted at each demonstration site: an introductory visit before the kickoff conference, a post-implementation visit in June 1999 at three to four months after the MTFs began implementing the guideline, and another visit in February 2000 (at month nine or ten of implementation).[1] During each post-implementation site visit, RAND staff members interviewed the MTF's implementation team and other individuals or groups involved or affected by introduction of practice changes in response to the new guideline. All groups were candid in reporting progress and identifying issues and problems they encountered. At the conclusion of each evaluation visit, we briefed the MTF command group about what we had learned and issues identified. Summary reports of the results of the

[1]Following the kickoff conference in November 1998, there was a delay of approximately four months before the sites began implementation actions for the low back pain guideline. The delay was due to time conflicts during the holidays as well as delays in completion of the practice guideline, metrics, and toolkit items. The sites had begun at least some implementation activities by April 1999.

second round of site visits for the four participating MTFs are presented in Appendix B. These reports document the status of the MTFs at essentially the end of their proactive implementation activities.

A second source of process evaluation information was monthly progress reports prepared by the participating MTFs and submitted to RAND. These reports provided valuable information on implementation progress over time, and they also served as a stimulus for action by both the MTFs and MEDCOM as the MTFs identified issues requiring resolution.

Finally, we developed brief questionnaires designed to assess the climate in the MTFs for guideline implementation, both at baseline and at the end of the demonstration, and to gather information from participants about their experiences in working with the guideline. Although the sample sizes were too small to be used for any rigorous statistical analysis, the completed questionnaires offered useful insights that we considered in developing our findings. The survey respondents were those most actively involved with the guideline, which could bias the surveys to be more optimistic regarding implementation progress. However, the broad distribution on survey responses within the same site suggests no major bias is present.

OUTCOME EVALUATION METHODS

An interrupted time series control-group design was used to assess the effects of the low back pain guideline demonstration. Quarterly administrative data on service utilization and medication prescriptions were collected for low back pain patients served by the demonstration and control sites. These data provided trend information both before and after introduction of the guideline in the Great Plains Region. The use of a control group allowed us to control for temporal trends that might be influencing observed effects. The design is represented in Table 2.1.

The six-month baseline period is October 1998 through March 1999, with the MTFs starting actions to implement the guideline in late March or early April 1999. Given that the kickoff conference was held

Table 2.1

Guideline Introduced (April 1999)

	Fiscal Year 1999				Fiscal Year 2000
Study Sites	1st Quarter	2nd Quarter	3rd Quarter	4th Quarter	1st Quarter
Demonstration MTFs	B	B	E	E	E
Control MTFs	C	C	C	C	C

NOTES: B = baseline, E = intervention for demonstration sites, and C = baseline condition for the control sites.

in November 1998, there was a four-month delay between the official start date of the conference and the initiation of actual implementation activities. This delay was due to several factors: the holiday season, delay by DoD and the VA in completing the practice guideline itself, and the time it took MEDCOM to provide the participating MTFs with the implementation tools and other support materials that had been identified at the conference. We designed the analysis of guideline effects to reflect the realities of this field experience.

Choice of Demonstration and Control Groups

The demonstration sites for this evaluation were the four low back pain guideline demonstration sites in the Great Plains Region. Two sets of MTFs were selected to serve as control sites:

- MTFs in the Great Plains Region that were introduced to the low back pain guideline but received no additional external assistance to facilitate implementation. Differences in performance between these MTFs and the demonstration MTFs yielded estimates of the extent to which the intensive implementation support activities provided during the demonstration contributed to implementation progress.
- MTFs located outside the Great Plains Region, which represent baseline trends in service and medication use for facilities that had no exposure to the low back pain guideline.

The peer groupings developed by the Army Patient Administration Systems and Biostatistical Activity (PASBA) were used to identify control MTFs that were similar to the demonstration MTFs in terms of size and service mix. In addition, the control sites outside the Great Plains Region were chosen to match sites included in the FMAS low back pain study performed for the National Quality Management Program, with the goal of facilitating combined analysis of the RAND data and FMAS chart abstraction data.

Data Sources

The analyses conducted in this study required data on outpatient visits, use of pain medications, and patient characteristics. Three DoD data systems were the sources of these data:

- Data on outpatient visits were obtained from the Standard Ambulatory Data Record (SADR) database extracted from MTF Ambulatory Data System (ADS) data.
- Prescription medications data were obtained from the Uniformed Services Prescription Database (USPD) maintained by the PharmacoEconomic Center (PEC). The earliest reliable data available were for the first quarter of fiscal year 1999 (FY99) (October–December 1999).
- Patient characteristics data were obtained from the Standard Installation/Division Personnel System (SIDPERS) database.

The SADR and USPD data were extracted by PASBA, and the SIDPERS data were extracted by the Center for Health Education and Studies (CHES); these extracted data files were transmitted to RAND for analysis. Details of the methods for extracting data from these sources and for construction of the analysis files are presented in Appendix A.

The Low Back Pain Population

The patient population for this study was limited to active duty Army personnel who received care for acute low back pain at one of the demonstration or control sites during the time period of the study. This design was selected because we could not obtain complete pharmaceutical data for all patients using these MTFs. At the time of the study, the only available pharmaceutical data were the MTF pharmacy data in the USPD. The USPD records provided reasonably complete data for active duty personnel because virtually all these personnel fill their prescriptions at MTF pharmacies. However, family members and retirees also use the National Mail Order Pharmacy or TRICARE retail pharmacies to fill some of their prescriptions, and we did not have access to these data.

The pharmacy data constraint was important because use of pain medications is a major aspect of care for acute low back pain patients, and one-half of the indicators selected for the study are measures of pain medication use. Even though this study is limited to active duty personnel, it provides useful information because acute low back pain is one of the major causes of lost duty days for this population. We encourage expansion of the analysis to also include family members and retirees as other service utilization and pharmaceutical data become available.

Indicators for Demonstration Effects

The indicators we defined to test effects of the low back pain practice guideline under demonstration conditions are listed in Table 2.2. These indicators measure the hypotheses regarding effects of using conservative treatment of acute low back pain, which are presented in Chapter One. The indicators are good choices for this demonstration because most of the participating MTFs focused their implementation actions on service delivery for acute low back pain (rather than chronic low back pain), so if observable effects occur, they are most likely to be for services delivered during the first six weeks of care.

These indicators are episode-based measures that encompass service use occurring within the six weeks following an initial patient visit for low back pain. The first three indicators address effects on service utilization with respect to physical therapy (PT) or manipulation services, follow-up primary care visits, or specialty care referrals. The remaining three indicators address use of pain medications, including muscle relaxants, narcotics, and NSAIDs.

A low back pain visit was defined as a visit with an ICD-9 diagnostic code of 722 (intervertebral disc disorders) or 724 (other and unspecified disorders of back) in any diagnosis code position (the SADR data have a total of four possible codes). An initial visit was defined as a low back pain visit to a physician, nurse practitioner, or physician assistant with no other low back pain visits in the previous 90 days. Any low back pain visits that occurred more than 90 days before the initial visit were assumed to pertain to a previous episode of care. Visits to physical therapy, clinical nursing, obstetrics, orthotics, and psychiatry were excluded because they were not considered to be initial visits, although some could be part of an episode of care.

A valid initial visit represented the start of an episode of low back pain care, and each episode of care was assigned to the quarter-year in which its initial visit occurred. Within each quarter, we tabulated

Table 2.2

Indicators Used to Measure Effects on Service Utilization Related to Implementation of the DoD/VA Low Back Pain Practice Guideline

	Calculation of the Indicator	
Indicator	Numerator	Denominator
Percentage of acute low back pain patients referred for PT or manipulation in first six weeks	Number of patients in the denominator who are referred to PT/manipulation in first six weeks	Number of patients with initial visits for low back pain
Percentage of acute low back pain patients referred to specialists in first six weeks of treatment	Number of patients in the denominator who are referred to specialists in first six weeks	Number of patients with initial visits for low back pain
Number of primary care visits per acute low back pain patient during first six weeks of treatment	Number of primary care visits for denominator in six weeks after first visit	Number of patients with initial visits for low back pain
Percentage of acute low back pain patients prescribed muscle relaxants in first six weeks of treatment	Number of patients in the denominator who were prescribed muscle relaxants in first six weeks	Number of patients with initial visits for low back pain
Percentage of acute low back pain patients prescribed narcotics in first six weeks of treatment	Number of patients in the denominator who were prescribed narcotics in first six weeks	Number of patients with initial visits for low back pain
Percentage of NSAID prescriptions that were for high-cost NSAIDs	Number of NSAID prescriptions in the denominator that were for high-cost NSAIDs	Number of NSAID prescriptions for low back pain patients in first six weeks

service-use counts for each indicator (visits or medication records) for the episodes starting in that quarter. Thus, trends over time were generated for each indicator, including each of two quarters preceding and three quarters following the introduction of the low back pain practice guideline. Definitions of these measures are described below.

Definition of Key Variables

Variables for service utilization and pain medications were derived for calculation of the indicators being analyzed. We also defined variables for the gender, age, and military rank of each patient with an episode of low back pain care in our analysis data files. These variables are summarized here, and additional coding details are provided in Appendix A.

Service Utilization. The measures of effects of the low back pain guideline demonstration included three types of service utilization: referrals to physical therapy or chiropractic care, follow-up primary care visits, and referrals to specialty care. These analyses used SADR outpatient encounter data. Only visits considered to be part of the low back pain episode of care were included in the analysis, as determined by diagnosis codes recorded for each encounter. For the physical therapy/chiropractic care visits and the follow-up primary care visits, all low back pain encounters were defined as relevant visits. For specialty care visits, we expanded the list of diagnosis codes to include other relevant conditions or complications associated with low back pain that might require specialty care (see Appendix A). We used the following coding to define each type of outpatient visit:

- *Physical therapy or manipulation visit*—a visit in a physical therapy clinic or "other" orthopedic clinic, or provided by a physical therapist (provider specialty code 706).
- *Primary care visit*—a visit in a family practice, primary care, flight medicine, or internal medicine clinic.
- *Neurology visit*—a visit in a neurology clinic or provided by a neurologist (specialty code 060).

- *Neurosurgery visit*—a visit in a neurosurgery clinic or provided by a neurosurgeon (specialty code 106).
- *Physical medicine and rehabilitation*—a visit in a physical medicine or pain management clinic or provided by a physical medicine physician (specialty code 090) or a physical medicine and rehabilitation physician (specialty code 950).
- *Orthopedics visit*—a visit in an orthopedics clinic or provided by an orthopedic surgeon (specialty code 140) or orthopedics physician (specialty code 947).
- *Specialty care visit*—a visit in a neurology, neurosurgery, physical medicine, or orthopedics clinic or provided by one of those specialty providers.

The number of visits for each type of service was tabulated for each episode of care. For physical therapy or manipulation visits, a dichotomous variable was coded for each episode, which was assigned a value of "1" if the episode had one or more visits or a value of "0" if there were no visits. The same coding was performed for specialty care visits. The variable used for the number of follow-up primary care visits in an episode was the actual count of visits.

Pain Medications. Working with the generic names of the drugs prescribed in the USPD records, we defined five groups of medications for the analysis of low back pain medication indicators: muscle relaxants, narcotics, high-cost NSAIDs, low-cost NSAIDs, and any NSAIDs. The specific drugs included in each medication group are listed in Appendix A. The number of prescriptions for each type of medication was tabulated for each episode of care. Similar to the variables used for the service utilization indicators, dichotomous variables were derived for each episode of care indicating whether or not the patient filled at least one prescription for muscle relaxants or narcotics during the episode. The analysis for high-cost NSAIDs was performed using two methods: coding of each episode for use of high-cost NSAIDs or not (episode-level data) and calculation of the percentage of NSAID prescriptions that were high-cost (using prescription-level data).

Patient Characteristics. Gender, age, and military rank were the patient characteristics used in the analysis, for which the source was

SIDPERS data. Patients were classified by military rank and by age using the following categories:

- *Patient age*—categories of age less than 30 years, 30 to 39 years, or 40 years or older.
- *Rank of active duty personnel*—officer (ranks of 20 to 29), warrant (ranks of 10 to 15), or enlisted (ranks of 1 to 9), based on coding in the SIDPERS data. An alternative variable was also defined that collapsed the officer and warrant officer rank into one officer category.

Analysis Methods

The first step in the analysis was to calculate each indicator for episodes in each quarter-year of the study period. For each measure, we then estimated the baseline performance for the MTFs, described quarterly trends for the demonstration and control sites, and tested the statistical significance of any observed differences in performance of the demonstration site compared with the control sites. See Appendixes A and C for details on the statistical tests.

Benchmarking. We combined data from the first and second quarter of FY99 to create baseline measures on the six indicators for the nine MTFs included in the study as either demonstration or control sites. For each indicator, we compared the performance of each MTF with the mean performance of all other MTFs combined (i.e., excluding the index MTF). The baseline performance information for the MTFs is reported in Chapter Three, including bar graphs with MTF comparisons for each of the six measures and testing of the statistical significance of differences among them in performance on each measure. We did not adjust for multiple comparisons, which can increase the probability of Type 1 errors (false negatives), but we report significance levels at both the 0.05 and 0.01 thresholds.

Descriptions of Trends for Indicators. To describe trend information, we prepared tables and graphs displaying estimates for the six indicators over the five quarter-year periods included in the study, aggregated separately for the demonstration and control sites. In many cases, we found substantial differences in performance levels or trends among the demonstration or control sites. We examined the effects of these differences on overall trends by describing trends separately for each demonstration site, or by describing aggregate trends for the relevant group of sites after excluding an MTF with outlying values. The quantitative results were compared with the implementation strategies of the demonstration sites to better interpret the observed trends. This step allowed us to assess the extent to which those strategies were reflected in observed service changes (or not). The results of these analyses are reported in Chapter Six.

Testing the Significance of Indicator Trends. The final step of the analysis was to test whether observed changes in service rates or medication use, if any, were large enough to be statistically significant after controlling for temporal trends and for patient characteristics. As described above, the control sites were included in the study to allow us to control for external trends that might be affecting use of services or medications for low back pain for all Army MTFs. For each of the six indicators, we estimated a regression model with the dependent variable being the indicator of interest and the predictor variables including a dichotomous variable for demonstration or control, a set of dummy variables for the quarter-year periods, and variables for the patient characteristics. To test for changes in the indicator for the demonstration sites between the baseline and intervention periods, we also included one or more interaction terms for demonstration sites and for each of the three quarters of the intervention period. To determine the final specification of the interaction terms, we were guided by the observed trends for the measures and the significance of the coefficients on the interaction term for each quarter. The results of the analysis are presented in Chapter Six, and the specification of each model and detailed results of the modeling are reported in Appendix C.

Chapter Three

BASELINE PERFORMANCE OF THE STUDY SITES

Baseline information on the performance of MTFs with respect to relevant key measures can be used to guide MTF strategies for implementing a practice guideline, including both the levels of performance and variation in performance across MTFs. In this chapter, we present this information for each of the six measures used as indicators of the effects of the demonstration on treatment for acute low back pain patients.

The baseline for the study was the six-month period preceding the date that the MTFs started implementation of the practice guideline, which was late March or early April 1999 (see Chapter Two for discussion of reasons for the delayed start of implementation). Thus, the baseline period included October 1998 through March 1999, the first six months of fiscal year 1999. We calculated average values for the indicators across this time period for each of the nine MTFs (the four demonstration sites and five control sites) included in the study. We also calculated an overall average value as a benchmark against which values for each of the MTFs were compared. These nine facilities represent approximately one-quarter of the Army MTFs.

These comparisons can be used to examine the extent of variation across facilities in provision of acute low back pain services and to highlight particular facilities or aspects of care that merit targeted intervention for strengthening practices. The direction provided by the DoD/VA low back pain guideline should be considered when interpreting the baseline performance data. As shown in Table 3.1, the guideline provides a "gold standard" for performance on muscle re-

Table 3.1

Interpretation of MTF Baseline Performance on the Low Back Pain Indicators

Indicator	Guideline Direction	Baseline MTF Performance Focus
Physical therapy/ manipulation	Evidence of beneficial effects not strong; clinical judgment regarding use.	Variation
Specialty referrals	After eliminating serious problems, try conservative treatment before referring; specialists report inappropriate referrals.	Variation
Number of primary care visits	After eliminating serious problems, try conservative treatment; could either reduce or increase primary care visits.	Variation
Use of muscle relaxants	No evidence that muscle relaxants help low back pain; advises they not be used.	Levels
Use of narcotics	Advises use of NSAIDs first; progressing to narcotics only if serious pain persists.	Variation
Use of high-cost NSAIDs	Guideline is silent on high-cost versus low-cost NSAIDs; PEC reports little difference in efficacy.	Variation

laxants, but it is less directive for the other indicators used in this study, allowing for clinical judgment or for variations in patterns of service related to differences among MTF capabilities or other factors. However, wide variation across MTFs on any given measure suggests that MTFs may not be providing care consistently, which could include overtreatment in some cases and undertreatment in others.

DISTRIBUTIONS OF MTFs ON LOW BACK PAIN MEASURES

Presented here is a series of figures (Figures 3.1 through 3.6) that display graphically the baseline performance of the study MTFs on the six indicators of low back pain care. The first bar on the left of each graph is the overall average baseline performance for all nine MTFs, and the remaining bars show the values for each of the nine MTFs. To protect the confidentiality of individual MTFs, the results are reported anonymously (Cs are control MTFs, and sites are demonstration sites).

We tested the statistical significance of the differences of MTF values by comparing each MTF's average value for a measure to the average value for the remaining eight MTFs. When the performance of an MTF differs significantly from the average of the other MTFs, the MTF's label in the legend is followed by asterisks (* for $p < 0.05$, ** for $p < 0.01$). As discussed in Chapter Two, both the clinical significance of observed differences among MTFs and the statistical significance of these differences should be considered when interpreting these results.

Figures 3.1 through 3.3 show the baseline performance of the nine MTFs on the three service utilization indicators. The referral rates for physical therapy or manipulation services were significantly lower than average for three MTFs and were significantly higher for three other MTFs (Figure 3.1). The remaining three MTFs did not differ significantly from the average.

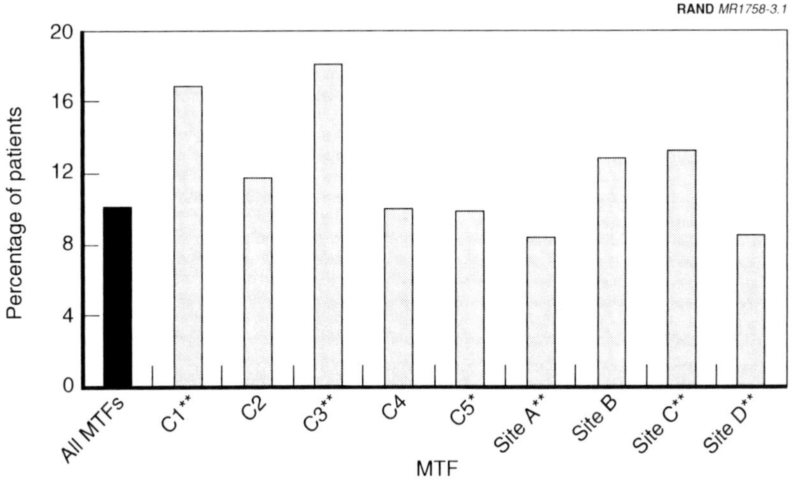

NOTES: To protect the confidentiality of individual MTFs, the results are reported anonymously (Cs are control MTFs, and sites are demonstration sites). * is for $p < 0.05$, and ** is for $p < 0.01$.

Figure 3.1—Baseline Percentages of Acute Low Back Pain Patients Referred for Physical Therapy or Manipulation Services Within Six Weeks of Initial Low Back Pain Encounter

The facilities varied widely in the number of follow-up primary care visits per episode of care, with all but two MTFs differing significantly from average. The MTFs with the lowest and highest rates of primary care visits differed by almost 80 percent (Figure 3.2). Referral rates to specialty care varied even more widely across MTFs. One MTF had an average rate that was 100 percent higher than the mean and another had a rate that was 50 percent lower. Differences from the mean were statistically significant for all MTFs (Figure 3.3).

Figures 3.4 through 3.6 show the baseline performance of the nine MTFs on the indicators for use of pain medications. An overall average of 50 percent of acute low back pain episodes treated by the nine MTFs had prescriptions for muscle relaxants. This rate compares with a rate of 35 percent of civilian patients being prescribed muscle relaxants found in a Seattle study (Cherkin et al., 1998). It also contrasts strongly to the guideline recommendation against any use of

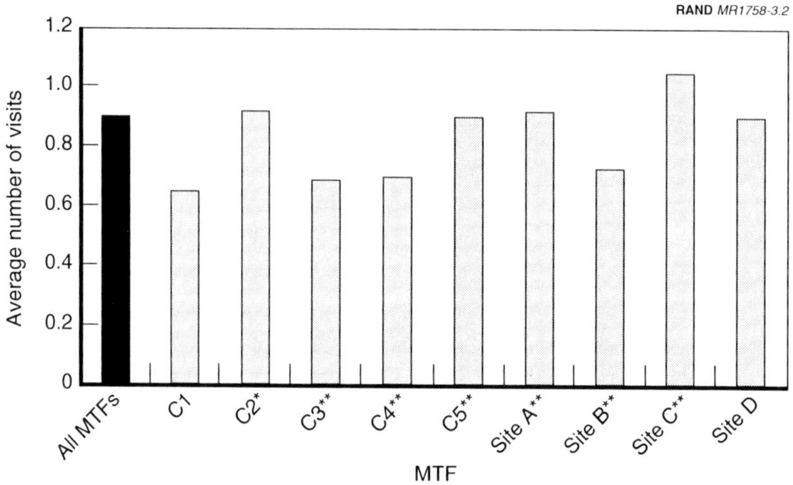

NOTES: To protect the confidentiality of individual MTFs, the results are reported anonymously (Cs are control MTFs, and sites are demonstration sites). * is for $p < 0.05$, and ** is for $p < 0.01$.

Figure 3.2—Baseline Average Number of Primary Care Visits for Acute Low Back Pain Patients Within Six Weeks of Initial Low Back Pain Encounter

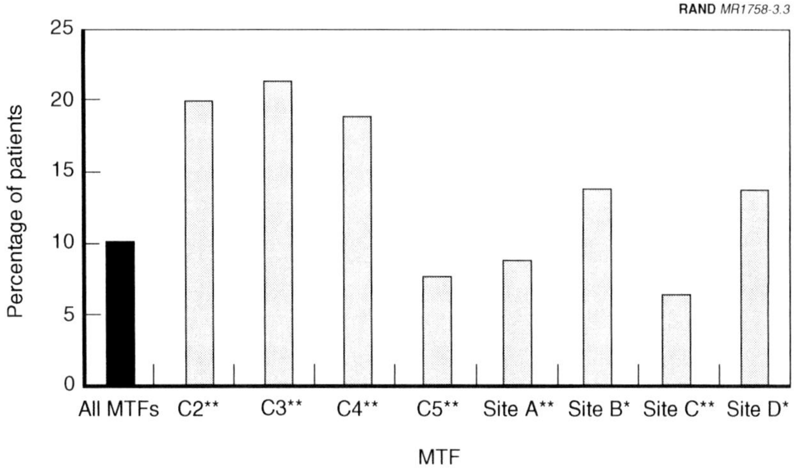

NOTES: To protect the confidentiality of individual MTFs, the results are reported anonymously (Cs are control MTFs, and sites are demonstration sites). * is for $p < 0.05$, and ** is for $p < 0.01$.

Figure 3.3—Baseline Percentages of Acute Low Back Pain Patients Referred for Specialty Care Services Within Six Weeks of Initial Low Back Pain Encounter

muscle relaxants. Rates of muscle relaxant use were significantly lower than the overall average for only two MTFs, while rates were significantly higher for five MTFs (Figure 3.4).

Narcotics were prescribed for about one-third of low back pain episodes overall. Two MTFs had significantly lower rates of narcotics use, and four had significantly higher rates (Figure 3.5). Finally, rates of prescription of high-cost NSAIDs were low, on average, but varied significantly across MTFs (Figure 3.6). Two MTFs had rates much higher than the average, and three MTF had rates that were only one-third lower than average.

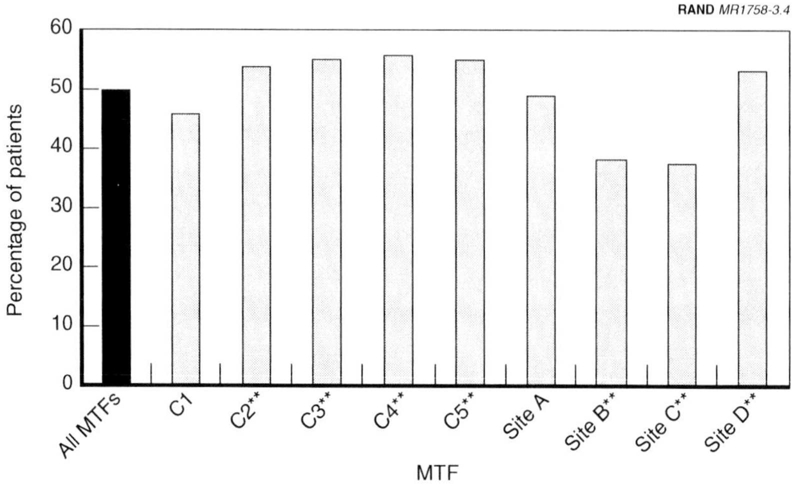

NOTES: To protect the confidentiality of individual MTFs, the results are reported anonymously (Cs are control MTFs, and sites are demonstration sites). * is for $p < 0.05$, and ** is for $p < 0.01$.

Figure 3.4—Baseline Percentages of Acute Low Back Pain Patients Prescribed Muscle Relaxant Medications Within Six Weeks of Initial Low Back Pain Encounter

DISCUSSION

Three distinct patterns emerge from the assessment of the baseline performance of the nine MTFs on each of the six indicators of care for low back pain patients. First, there is substantial variation among the MTFs in the rates of use for physical therapy/manipulation services, primary care visits, and specialty referrals. Second, there are consistently high percentages of patients prescribed muscle relaxants or narcotic pain relievers, neither of which are recommended by the guideline because scientific evidence does not support their use for acute low back pain. Third, providers at a few MTFs appear to be using high-cost NSAIDs for their patients at high rates compared with the other MTFs, although the overall rate of use is low (an average of 4 percent of patients used high-cost NSAIDs across all MTFs).

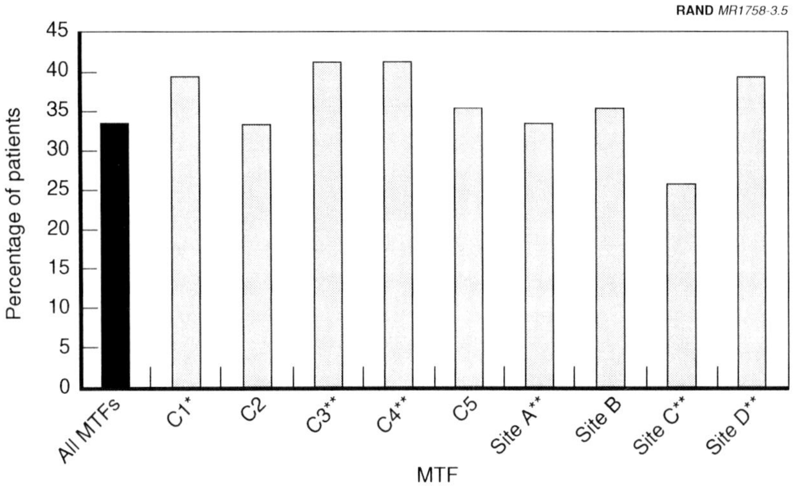

NOTES: To protect the confidentiality of individual MTFs, the results are reported anonymously (Cs are control MTFs, and sites are demonstration sites). * is for $p < 0.05$, and ** is for $p < 0.01$.

Figure 3.5—Baseline Percentages of Acute Low Back Pain Patients Prescribed Narcotic Medications Within Six Weeks of Initial Low Back Pain Encounter

These observed patterns are good examples of how baseline data can be used to assess current practices and begin to identify priority issues on which finite resources can be focused. For example, a priority clearly could be placed on reducing use of muscle relaxants by working with providers to change their prescribing methods. This is a particularly good example because there is such strong scientific evidence against using muscle relaxants, and providers are prescribing them for one-half of the patients in the study sample.

The wide variation across MTFs for the three service use indicators raises the question, What is the desired rate of use, for which there is no real "gold standard?" However, MTFs with unusually high or low rates should assess why they differ so much from others, which may lead to identification of quality issues that can be corrected.

RAND MR1758-3.6

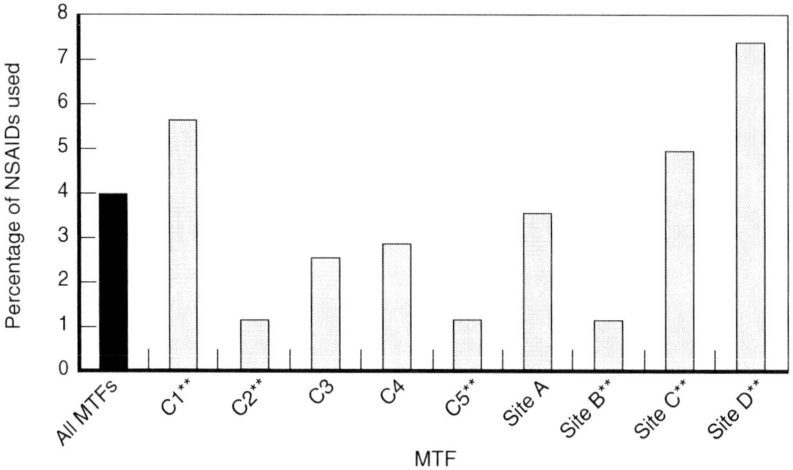

NOTES: To protect the confidentiality of individual MTFs, the results are reported anonymously (Cs are control MTFs, and sites are demonstration sites). * is for $p < 0.05$, and ** is for $p < 0.01$.

Figure 3.6—Baseline Use of High-Cost NSAIDs by Acute Low Back Pain Patients as a Percentage of All NSAIDs Used

When considering these results, we note that a statistically significant departure from a mean score for a measure is important only if an MTF's performance on the measure is far enough away from the mean to be clinically important. For example, an MTF may have a baseline rate of physical therapy referrals that is 50 percent higher than the mean but remains in the realm of clinical appropriateness. Conversely, the use rate for muscle relaxants for the MTF with the lowest rate may still be too high, which would also be cause for concern.

Chapter Four

INFRASTRUCTURE FOR GUIDELINE IMPLEMENTATION

The implementation teams at the demonstration MTFs were responsible for working with MTF primary care clinics to introduce practices recommended by the guideline for low back pain management, but they were not expected to carry out these changes alone. MEDCOM and RAND provided instructions to the MTFs regarding the organization of the MTF implementation teams and activities, encompassing both support by the MTF command and a clear focus of leadership and membership for the implementation teams. MEDCOM also made a commitment to provide corporate support in the form of policy guidance regarding recommended practices, tools and materials for MTF use in implementing those practices, and monitoring of progress in achieving new practices.

In this chapter, we report our findings regarding the infrastructure established for the low back pain guideline demonstration. We first describe the MEDCOM support structure and activities. Then we describe the MTF support structure, including support by the MTF command team and roles of the guideline champions, facilitators, and implementation teams.

MEDCOM SUPPORT

The corporate responsibility for operating the AMEDD program for evidence-based practice guidelines was assigned to the MEDCOM Quality Management Directorate. Initially, the staff for this new initiative consisted of a full-time program director and a secretary. This office was under strong pressure to begin the low back pain demonstration, and to follow it quickly with additional guideline demonstrations. As a result, the staff were managing multiple tasks in a rapidly evolving initiative. By the end of the low back pain guideline demonstration (the time of our second round of site visits), the asthma guideline demonstration had begun and preparations were under way for kicking off the diabetes guideline demonstration. The MEDCOM program staff had also been expanded by then, with two full-time guideline representatives to support MTFs in implementing these demonstrations as well as other guidelines planned to be introduced.

The low back pain guideline demonstration involved a steep learning curve by all participants because it was the first one conducted by the new MEDCOM program, and methods and support mechanisms were being identified and evolving in real time as the demonstration progressed. The MEDCOM staff were committed and highly motivated, and they worked collaboratively with the MTF teams in these development efforts. As they were learning "on the job" lessons, the program staff were simultaneously preparing for subsequent demonstrations. As a result, the development and coordination of program components and toolkit materials for the low back pain demonstration took longer than initially planned.

The MEDCOM staff supported the MTFs in implementing the low back pain guideline by (1) organizing an off-site kickoff conference to introduce the implementation teams to the guideline and help them develop implementation action plans, (2) providing the MTFs with a toolkit of items to support guideline implementation, and (3) encouraging communications and technical support among the demonstration sites and MEDCOM. We describe our findings regarding each of these components.

The Kickoff Conference

The implementation teams gathered for two days on November 19–20, 1998, in San Antonio, Texas, to prepare for implementation of the low back pain guideline in their respective MTFs. Upon arrival at the conference, participants were given a notebook containing information on the guideline, toolkit items, and instructions for preparing an implementation action plan. The conference began with a half-day plenary session at which the low back pain guideline was introduced and instructions for action plan development were provided. For the remainder of the conference, each team met in a separate room to prepare strategies and action plans for implementing the guideline at each facility. Each MTF team had designated a facilitator who guided the team through a planning process developed by RAND. The product of that process was an implementation action plan that included goals, an overall strategy, sets of detailed actions for practice changes, and metrics for monitoring progress in implementation. The MTF teams briefed the commander of the Great Plains Region on their action plans at the end of the conference.

Because of the pressure to get into the field, the demonstration was scheduled to begin before the final DoD/VA low back pain guideline document was completed and could be disseminated to the participating MTFs. The guideline presented to MTF teams at the kickoff conference was a draft version, and the final document did not become available until late January 1999. This issue contributed to delays in educating team members and providers on the contents of the practice guideline, as well as to some loss of credibility for MEDCOM.

Participants were asked to evaluate the usefulness of the conference and to make suggestions for improvements. Participants reported they found the planning activities to be useful. They also thought that holding the conference off site, away from day-to-day activities, allowed them to focus effectively on their planning tasks. To improve the kickoff conference, participants suggested that preparatory materials be sent to the MTFs ahead of the conference and that more emphasis be placed on practical application of the guidelines. These suggestions were incorporated into the demonstrations for implementing the asthma and diabetes guidelines. Also, RAND considered this feedback as it prepared a revised implementation guide, adding a sample action plan for the low back pain guideline and specific examples of effective implementation actions (see Nicholas et al., 2001).

The Low Back Pain Toolkit

In preparation for the low back pain guideline demonstration, MEDCOM and CHPPM had prepared a draft form for documenting care to low back pain patients and a draft patient education brochure. The concept of a comprehensive toolkit to support guideline implementation actually surfaced spontaneously at the end of the demonstration kickoff conference. Participants were enthusiastically supportive of centralized development of tools, which they felt would be a higher quality and less costly alternative to each MTF developing the same materials itself. Since this first demonstration, MEDCOM has prepared toolkits for all practice guidelines implemented by the Army.

Based on suggestions from the conference participants, MEDCOM and CHPPM developed several toolkit materials and made them available to the MTFs in January through March 1999. The MTF teams delayed the start of their implementation actions while they waited for these tools, which led to a loss of momentum in some facilities. As the various toolkit items became available, the sites incorporated them into their activities (see Table 4.1).

Feedback from the sites on the toolkit items was sought during our first evaluation site visits, and MEDCOM and CHPPM made revisions to the tools in response to that feedback. The revised tools became available to the MTFs at various times during the demonstration, as noted above. By our second site visit, the MTFs had received all the revised items except the encounter documentation form 695-R.

Documentation Form 695-R. This documentation form included a section to be filled out by the clinic staff, a section for the patient to complete, and a section to be completed by the physician. At our first

Table 4.1

Tools Developed for the Low Back Pain Guideline Toolkit

Toolkit Items	Date Completed	Date Revised
Encounter documentation form	January 1999	March 2000
Provider education videotape	January 1999	April 1999
Guideline key elements cards		
Desktop 8 1/2 x 11" card	February 1999	—
Pocket-sized card	February 2000	—
Patient education materials		
Written pamphlet	March 1999	—
Videotape	January 1999	May 1999

site visits, primary care providers generally liked the form, but they felt it did not fully meet their needs. They suggested the following changes to the form itself:

- Increase the space available to write in.
- Add a stick figure to show location of pain.
- Add boxes for referrals for CT scans and back pain management classes.
- Add space to record results of lab tests.

Several issues arose over time that discouraged use of the form by providers, especially those who were already predisposed against using new forms. Ultimately, the form was used only sporadically by the demonstration sites. The form was intended to be completed for each clinic visit by patients with low back pain. Although physicians thought the form was well-suited for the initial visit, they felt it was too long for follow-up visits and suggested that a shorter form be developed for those visits. They also thought the form was poorly suited for patients with multiple diagnoses, who represent a significant share of their cases.

Ancillary staff at the demonstration sites indicated that the patient portion of the form was time consuming to fill out and that the language used was above the reading level of their patients. They suggested patient material be written at the third-grade reading level. They also requested that the patient section of the form be available in other languages (Spanish, Korean, and German) because many patients did not read or speak English. (The patients for whom they were using the guideline were all patients using the participating clinics, not just active duty personnel that were the sample for the effects analysis.)

Based on the suggestions made during our first round of site visits, the encounter form was revised by MEDCOM and CHPPM staff, in consultation with the MTF champions and selected team members. However, it took in excess of eight months to complete and disseminate the revised documentation form. By the time of our second visit, the sites had received the revised forms, but the team leaders had not yet distributed copies to providers and clinic staff. Hence, we could not verify the sites' assessment of the revised form, and it remains to be seen whether the revisions made will encourage use of the form in the future.

Provider Education Videotape. The first continuing medical education (CME) video developed to introduce primary care providers to the guideline was not well received. The video contained a step-by-step review of the low back pain guideline and a demonstration of a straight-leg-raise test, which providers rated positively. However, they thought the video was geared too much to specialists and contained unnecessary material.

A revised CME video was designed specifically for primary care providers. Although the new video was produced quickly (less than three months), the sites received the new video after they had completed their first round of provider education sessions. None of the sites had conducted a second round of education sessions by the time of our second site visits, so we could not assess the value of the new video to them.

Guideline Key Elements Cards. The sites had not yet received the desktop and pocket cards containing the algorithms and key elements of the guideline as of the time of our first site visits. At our second site visits, the MTF teams indicated the cards were valuable reminders, especially for physician assistants (PAs), young physicians, and physicians who do not see low back pain patients frequently. Overall, physicians rated these cards as "good" to "very good."

Patient Education Materials. The pamphlet providing patient education on low back pain became available in several languages as of March 1999. The brochure was praised by nearly everyone including primary care providers, ancillary staff, and patients. The sites have distributed the pamphlet extensively to patients.

By contrast, the first patient education video was not well received by the MTF teams, and MEDCOM provided a replacement video. Only a few staff had seen the new video at the time of our site visits, but they rated it as "very good." Use of the patient video was hampered by constraints in the physical layouts of clinics and troop medical clinics (TMCs) and the lack of appropriate equipment. Only one MTF actually used the video for patient education.

Addition to the Toolkit: Standard Profile Form. At the first round of site visits, some staff indicated they would like to have available a standard profile form that specified the set of duty restrictions appropriate for acute low back pain. A profile form had been developed by one of the demonstration sites, which MEDCOM adopted and included in the toolkit of materials for the low back pain guideline. However, this form was not widely distributed at the sites and only about one-third of physicians we interviewed had seen or used it. Those who had seen it rated it as "good."

Several other new toolkit items were suggested by the sites, including a standard "back class education" model, training material for nurses and administrative staff, and wall posters containing the key elements of the guideline. A few of these suggestions had been acted upon by MEDCOM as of the second round of site visits.

Information Exchange

Several information exchange mechanisms were considered to help the MTFs share their implementation experiences and learn from each other. These included email and web-based systems as well as periodic audio and videoconferences. We saw value in testing a variety of techniques, which would reinforce messages and information sharing and also would allow us to learn which techniques are most useful for the participants.

Listserve Options. An electronic listserve can be established as a free-standing email system or as part of a web-based bulletin board. With an email-based listserve, the participants are signed up as members and can exchange email with all other members by addressing a single message to the listserve's email address. The listserve can also be linked to a web-based home site with a bulletin board and chat rooms.

Participants at the low back pain kickoff conference were asked to complete a brief survey on their current use of electronic media (email and the web) and their interest in various listserve features. The results of the survey indicated that it would be important to use email for communications among the sites at the time of the demonstration. Almost three-quarters of the demonstration team members reported they had regular access to an email system, but fewer than

10 percent had regular access to the web. Of those with email access, almost 85 percent used email frequently. By contrast, only 37 percent of those with web access used it frequently. Almost two-thirds of the participants reported they would prefer to use an email system for communications during the demonstration. Additional written comments on the survey form revealed a desire for a fast, easy-to-use system and raised some concerns about limitations of the current capabilities of their systems.

A home site for the low back pain demonstration was set up on the AMEDD Knowledge Management Network (KMN) immediately following the kickoff conference. KMN is an Army-wide electronic system used primarily for educational purposes. It was chosen over a simpler email listserve because the AMEDD's leadership preferred to use existing capabilities to support implementation of guidelines whenever possible. Each individual had to register on the network before being able to use KMN. Registration involved a lengthy series of steps, and most who tried to register found the process complex and confusing. In the end, few demonstration participants chose to register, and even fewer (five to ten) actually used the system. KMN did not provide the user-friendly communication mechanism hoped for, and it ended up not being used. Later attempts to replace it with a dedicated listserve were also unsuccessful due to technical difficulties. Hence, the demonstration proceeded without an electronic means for quick communications across sites and between sites and MEDCOM.

Academic Detailing (Technical Support). MEDCOM used periodic teleconferences or videoconferences to communicate with the sites during the demonstration. MEDCOM staff also participated in the two rounds of site visits for the RAND evaluation, during which they were able to address questions from the sites and more generally assist them in their implementation activities. However, as discussed above, the small MEDCOM staff team was being pulled in multiple directions to start up the low back pain demonstration and also to prepare for implementation of the asthma and diabetes guidelines. As a result, MEDCOM was less responsive than needed, and some sites ran out of supplies and lacked instructions for reordering them.

STRUCTURE AND SUPPORT AT THE MTFs

To prepare for implementation of the low back pain guideline, commanders of the MTFs participating in the demonstration were requested to appoint a multidisciplinary implementation team of eight to ten individuals who represented the mix of clinical and support staff involved in delivering care for patients with low back pain. The responsibility of the implementation team was to develop an action plan and facilitate its implementation. In addition, the commanders were requested to designate a *guideline champion* and a *facilitator* to lead the implementation activities. The champion was the leader of the implementation activities and the MTF team. Preferably, this individual was a primary care physician who was an opinion leader and had a strong commitment to the successful implementation of the guideline. The facilitator was to guide the implementation team in developing an implementation action plan and then to provide support to the champion and team in coordinating and managing the implementation process. This individual needed experience facilitating group decisionmaking processes as well as to be able to organize work processes and to work with data for quality management and monitoring activities.

Command Support and Accountability

Commanders at the demonstration MTFs had agreed to participation in the low back pain guideline demonstration. Over the life of the demonstration, however, the support of the MTF commanders ranged from moderately strong to absent, and some commanders appeared to be ambivalent or passive toward the guideline work. Changes in command occurred at two sites during the demonstration. This change did not alter the positive (but still passive) command support of the guideline at one MTF. The new commander at the other MTF had yet to be briefed or see a copy of the low back pain guideline by the time of our second visit.

All the commanders designated guideline champions, facilitators, and implementation teams, and they authorized the teams' participation in the two-day off-site conference that initiated the demonstration. When implementation activities began, none of the participating MTFs provided the leaders and members of the implementation team with dedicated time to devote uniquely to carrying out the guideline action plan. Team members continued to be responsible for their existing job functions, and time spent on actions to implement the low back pain guideline was added to those responsibilities. Nor did MTF commands request regular reporting, and hence, accountability, on implementation progress. Indeed, at one site, the commander gave the explicit signal that implementation of the guideline was not a priority for him, and staff acted accordingly, undertaking virtually no actions to introduce new practices for managing low back pain patients.

Climate survey results reinforce these observations of weak command support. Implementation team members responding to the RAND survey perceived that complying with implementation would not reap rewards for them and failing to comply would have no adverse consequences. Two out of every three respondents said there would be a "good" to "very good" chance that a staff member would be noticed if she or he did not cooperate with guideline implementation, but an overwhelming majority (94 percent) of respondents indicated they had "no risk" or "slight risk" if they did not cooperate. Similarly, a majority of respondents indicated that there was "no" to "little" chance that management would praise a staff member for cooperation with the guideline.

The Champions

The participating MTFs varied widely in their initial choices of champions to lead the low back pain guideline implementation activities, and the champions changed during the demonstration period. Three of the sites initially designated primary care physicians as champions, and the fourth site designated a specialist. All were clearly respected by their colleagues, and with one exception, they were committed to the successful implementation of the guideline. At some of the sites, the champions played more passive roles while the facilitators took on greater leadership roles. The champions reported that lack of "protected time" allocated for implementation of the guideline hampered their ability to be available and effective in leading implementation actions. They estimated that about one-third of their work time was needed for the first few months to perform this role effectively, but most were unable to do so.

At two sites, the champions did not change during the demonstration, which provided continuity of leadership. At another site, the first champion was a colonel and was replaced by a newly arrived captain (several ranks below colonel). This change effectively downgraded the role of the champion, such that the new champion (who was committed to the role) was unable to achieve desired practice changes. A similar change occurred at the last site, where the champion was replaced by a younger, lower-ranked physician. These changes reflected the low commitment at the two facilities to improvement of practices for treatment of low back pain.

The Facilitators

The demonstration MTFs selected individuals with a variety of backgrounds to serve as facilitators, supporting the MTF teams in their planning and execution of implementation actions. One of the MTFs did not designate a separate facilitator—the champion took on this role. For the remaining MTFs, one designated a military person as facilitator, one had a team of two facilitators (one military and one civilian), and the third had a civilian facilitator. The facilitators for these three MTFs were in staff positions in the MTF quality management or utilization management offices. The facilitators at two MTFs played active leadership roles throughout the demonstration, working in partnership with the champions to guide their teams in development of action plans, facilitating implementation activities, and generating data to monitor progress in carrying out the actions. One facilitator played a more supportive role to the guideline champion, who took the lead for the implementation actions.

The Implementation Teams

MEDCOM and RAND advised the MTFs to establish multidisciplinary implementation teams with 8 to 11 members, which has been shown to be an optimal size for effective team operation. Three of the MTFs complied with this guidance, establishing teams with 10 or 11 members. One of these sites later reduced its team to seven members after finding the team was too large to function effectively and it did not have the right mix of disciplines. The fourth MTF chose to use a 19-member team because the MTF wanted to include representatives from the multiple TMCs on post that served active duty personnel, to enhance buy-in for implementation at the TMCs. Although the large team size made it more difficult for the team to develop its action plan, later events suggest that this decision fulfilled the goal of encouraging TMC participation.

With few exceptions, the MTF teams included the clinical and support staff appropriate to the implementation of the low back pain guideline: primary care providers, physical therapists, ancillary staff, and utilization management/quality management (UM/QM) staff. They also all included representation from the TMCs where active duty personnel typically are first seen and treated. Some teams also included representation from the emergency department, occupational health, or the pharmacy. None of the sites included orthopedic, chiropractic, or neurosurgery specialists on its implementation team. The membership of the teams remained remarkably constant during the 15 months between the demonstration kickoff conference and our last visit. Members reported that command gave them a high level of autonomy to determine the actions, procedures, and schedule to implement the guideline.

In spite of staff continuity and autonomy, members of the implementation teams were only minimally involved in the actual implementation of the low back pain guideline. Teams at two of the sites had not met in six months. The sites gave various reasons for this low level of involvement. Team members were not able to allocate adequate time to fully participate in the work of the team. At sites with many TMCs and clinics, communications among team members and scheduling of meetings also proved difficult. On our survey at the second round of site visits, team members gave the lowest rating on issues related to the team activities to the "ability (of team members) to allocate adequate time for team activities." The next lowest rating from team members was given to the statement that "the team's overall performance had met their expectations."

LESSONS LEARNED

MEDCOM Support

- Development and implementation of a clinical practice guideline is a major undertaking requiring a significant commitment of staff resources. Having chosen to provide proactive corporate support to the Army MTFs for their practice guideline implementation activities, MEDCOM needs to commit resources and maintain staffing commensurate to the task.[1] As more guidelines are introduced and implementation activities mature, the roles and priorities of the MEDCOM staff should evolve to meet changing needs.

- Everything needed by the MTFs for effective implementation of a practice guideline should be in place before they are expected to begin working with the guideline. The relevant DoD/VA guideline should be completed and available for use, and associated metrics for monitoring progress should be established. In addition, MEDCOM should complete preparation and pilot testing of the materials included in the guideline toolkit.
- The design of the toolkit materials and other items to support the guideline should be responsive to the needs and preferences of the users. Intensive testing of the tools with a small number of MTFs before introducing them systemwide is an investment that can yield greater acceptance of the tools and more effective progress in improving practices.
- To maintain effective communications among MEDCOM and the MTFs on guideline implementation activities, MEDCOM will need to provide continuing leadership and communication mechanisms. This demonstration showed (as did subsequent demonstrations) that daily demands on the time of MTF staff impede their ability and willingness to take the initiative to communicate with other MTFs. Thus, any mechanisms established for cross-MTF communications should be easy to access and use, avoiding barriers that might further constrain communication activities.

---

[1]In spring 2000, the Army Surgeon General approved the establishment of the Condition/Guideline Management Program, which included an increase in staffing. The program is responsible for implementing up to 15 clinical practice guidelines across the Army treatment facilities over the next four to five years (unpublished RAND research by Georges Vernez et al. on the proposed managerial structure to support Army-wide implementation of clinical practice guidelines).

Support at the MTF

- MTF command support needs to be visible and proactive to make it clear that the leadership has placed a priority on achieving the best practices delineated in the practice guideline. This support involves both clear statements of support and provision of appropriate resources for a time-limited implementation period when the champion, facilitator, and implementation team are educating staff and introducing changes to clinical practices.
- Regular briefings should be scheduled by the MTF command to be updated on progress in carrying out the action plan, and administrative support should be provided to ensure that desired changes take place and to resolve issues that arise. As further reinforcement, the command should establish rewards and consequences for staff based on the extent to which they contribute to effective implementation of the new practices.
- The MTF guideline champion should be a physician who is motivated to lead the process of changing practices according to the practice guideline. This individual should be a respected opinion leader among the providers, with military rank commensurate to those of his or her peers at the MTF.
- The champion should be allocated protected time to provide the needed clinical leadership and time commitment to the implementation activities, especially during the startup period. The champion should also have the authority to make required procedural and clinical practice changes.
- Additional consideration should be given to the role and composition of the MTF implementation team. In this demonstration, there was substantial variation in the extent to which members of the implementation team participated in implementation activities. While the champion and facilitator are clearly the key players in carrying out the actions specified in the action plans, the strategic involvement of other team members contributes to building ownership in the implementation process and support for the new practices. For optimal results, the individuals given responsibility for carrying out specific actions in the plan should indeed be the ones with primary responsibility for the area addressed in those actions. Regular meetings of the implementa-

tion team may be useful for some MTFs but less desirable for others. However, an agreed-upon mechanism should be established for regular communications among the team members for strategic thinking, troubleshooting, and assessment of progress.

Chapter Five

IMPLEMENTATION ACTIONS BY THE DEMONSTRATION SITES

The low back pain guideline demonstration tested an implementation approach that included actions at both the corporate (MEDCOM) and local (MTF) levels. MEDCOM defined the desired clinical practices (as specified in the DoD/VA practice guideline) and key metrics to measure attainment of those practices, and it also provided several tools to assist the MTFs as they introduced new practices in response to the guideline. The practice changes were carried out by the MTFs, as the health care delivery organizations, and the MTFs were offered the flexibility to define strategies and clinical process changes within the context of their respective missions, populations, and administrative and clinical assets. Because these characteristics differed across facilities, we expected to observe differences among the MTFs' implementation strategies and the pace at which they introduced practice changes. We assessed the merits of this flexible approach in the evaluation, looking at how it affected the MTFs' ability to achieve best practices and progress toward consistent practices across facilities.

We report in this chapter the findings of the process evaluation with respect to the strategies and actions undertaken by the MTFs to implement best practices for management of low back pain patients. First, we summarize what we learned about the environment and climate for guideline implementation at the participating MTFs, which represent the settings within which the MTF teams were carrying out actions to modify the way the MTFs provide care to low back pain patients. Then we describe the strategies and actions the MTF teams identified in their implementation action plans and the progress they made in achieving desired practice changes. Finally, we summarize the lessons learned from the experiences of the MTFs participating in this demonstration.

THE MTF ENVIRONMENT

The four demonstration MTFs varied in their sizes and clinical capabilities as well as in their previous experience with quality improvement strategies and use of clinical practice guidelines. These features influenced the strategies chosen by the MTF teams for implementing the low back pain guideline and the actions they undertook to carry out the strategies. We summarize these features here. They are also taken into account in our assessment of implementation progress by the various sites.

MTF Service Capabilities

All the sites had the basic clinical capabilities for the treatment of low back pain including primary care clinics and physical therapy services. For three of the sites, primary care services were reasonably centralized at either hospital-based clinics or TMCs that were located separately. Two of these sites had two clinics and one TMC, and the other had two clinics and three TMCs. The fourth site had two clinics at the hospital and a network of seven TMCs located remotely across the post. All the MTFs had a mixture of contract and military physicians providing primary care services, but one of them reported being particularly dependent on contract providers. All sites indicated they had low ratios of ancillary support staff to providers, typically not exceeding one-to-one. Support staff limitations were a constraint on the MTFs' ability to take on new workload for implementing new practices.

The MTFs differed in the on-site availability of other relevant services, including relevant specialty clinics—physical medicine and rehabilitation, orthopedics, neurology, and neurosurgery. For specialty services they did not provide, the MTFs had access to the services from other MTFs or from community providers. Two sites offered back classes (for back pain management) at their wellness centers. In addition, two sites were participating in the Army chiropractic demonstration, and so chiropractic services were also available for low back pain patients.

Inherent to the Army environment are annual rotations and deployments of active duty personnel, including medical personnel. The sites varied in the frequency of deployments that took place during the demonstration. Two sites are the home bases of troops who deploy frequently. These sites experienced their typically high pace of deployments during the low back pain demonstration, including loss of some MTF providers to deployments.

Climate for Guideline Implementation

Among the factors that influence the extent to which a treatment facility achieves lasting improvements in its clinical care processes is the conduciveness of the organizational climate for guideline implementation. Relevant factors include the attitudes of key stakeholders regarding practice guidelines, their motivation for using guidelines, the nature of corporate cultures, and the priority that has been placed on quality improvement activities. If the MTF baseline operating climate is supportive, it should be easier for the implementation team to carry out its action plan and achieve desired effects on health care delivery and outcomes. Previous experience with clinical practice guidelines should also aid progress. Two sites had previous experience with guidelines.

At the start of the demonstration, we collected data on the baseline climates of the four MTFs in the demonstration, asking the members of the MTF command teams and guideline teams to complete a survey containing well-established measures of motivation and attitudes toward quality improvement and health care corporate culture. The climate survey consisted of five modules that addressed motivation for guideline implementation, supportiveness of climate, attitudes toward practice guidelines, hospital culture, and efforts to improve quality of care. Each module contained sets of items that respondents completed using scaled responses, and these items were summarized to obtain overall scores for each climate component. Selected components of this survey were administered again during the second round of post-implementation site visits at the end of the process evaluation, which allowed us to assess the extent to which changes in climate occurred during the demonstration.

As indicated in Table 5.1, the MTFs embarked on the low back pain guideline demonstration with a high level of commitment to quality improvement and with internal corporate environments that tended to encourage quality improvement activities. Attitudes toward practice guidelines were also generally positive, with MTF command staff generally more positive than members of the implementation teams. There were also statistically significant variations in attitudes among the sites.

A motivation measure was derived for each implementation team member based on the concept that team members will be motivated to initiate guideline activities when they perceive that (1) their efforts will lead to successful guideline implementation, (2) successful implementation will lead to improved job performance, and (3) improved job performance will be instrumental in achieving desired outcomes (e.g., career progress and improved patient outcomes).

Separate average scores were calculated for individual motivation and clinic/MTF motivation, as well as for a combined average score for overall motivation, measured as percentages of the maximum possible scores. The individual and combined motivation scores for the four MTFs, shown in Table 5.2, varied from less than 60 percent

Table 5.1

Baseline Survey Scores on Quality Improvement, MTF Climate, and Attitudes Toward Practice Guidelines

	Means (Standard Deviations) for Views on Quality Activities			
Respondent Group	Importance of Improving Quality of Care (range, 8 to 40)	MTF Current Status in Quality Improvement (range, 8 to 40)	MTF Climate for Guideline Implementation (range, 7 to 28)	Attitude Toward Practice Guidelines (range, 6 to 42)
All four MTFs				
Command teams	35.3 (3.7)	31.5 (6.3)	19.1 (4.0)*	35.0 (5.0)*
Implementation teams	35.4 (3.6)	33.4 (7.8)	17.1 (3.3)*	30.4 (5.8)*
Combined by MTF				
Site A	35.1 (3.9)	35.3 (6.7)	17.9 (3.6)	29.5 (6.9)*
Site B	34.2 (3.0)	30.3 (5.8)	16.5 (2.5)	32.5 (4.5)*
Site C	36.0 (3.4)	33.8 (6.9)	18.5 (3.8)	35.1 (5.0)*
Site D	36.5 (3.4)	30.4 (9.7)	17.2 (3.3)	31.0 (4.4)*

*Difference is significant at $p < 0.05$.

Table 5.2

Baseline Motivation for Guideline Implementation by the Implementation Teams

	Percentage of Maximum Scores for Perceptions of Motivation by the Guideline Implementation Teams		
Military Treatment Facility	Individual Motivation	Clinic/MTF Motivation	Combined Motivation
Site A	63.7	64.5	64.1
Site B	60.8	61.6	61.2
Site C	56.7	59.6	58.4
Site D	71.8	72.2	71.8

NOTES: The index scores have a maximum possible range of values from 1 to 245. The results reported are expressed as a percentage of the maximum score of 245. Differences among the MTFs are not statistically significant.

to over 70 percent of the maximum possible score. These differences were not statistically significant, in part because of the small numbers of respondents from each MTF.

The climate survey results indicate that the MTF implementation teams embarked on the low back pain guideline demonstration with a commitment to quality improvement and with internal corporate environments that tended to support guideline implementation efforts. Yet at the start of the demonstration, the MTF teams appeared to be only moderately positive in their attitudes toward practice guidelines and their motivation to use them to bring about desired quality improvements. These views could reflect a combination of some natural resistance by clinicians to the concept of practice guidelines, the uncertainty of participating in the demonstration, and concerns about increased workload. When combined with survey data (discussed in Chapter Four) in which participants said they would not be at risk if they did not cooperate, these results signify that obtaining and maintaining ongoing staff support for use of the guideline could be difficult.

IMPLEMENTATION ACTIVITIES AND PROGRESS

Implementation of the low back pain guideline was scheduled to begin within a month after the implementation teams had returned from the kickoff conference. However, there were delays in completing the guideline and toolkit materials, and as a result, the sites did not begin implementation until four months after the kickoff conference had been held. The result of this delay was a loss of momentum because the sites could not continue the pace of activity they had started at the conference. Below, we describe the demonstration sites' implementation strategies and activities, and we discuss the factors that appear to have affected their progress.

Implementation Strategies

At the kickoff conference, the teams were encouraged to approach implementation by undertaking actions on a small scale first, through which they could gain experience and correct problems identified before launching a major change in practices across the organization. One site used this approach when providers expressed concerns that using the low back pain documentation form would increase their workload. The site tested use of the form with two physicians at one TMC. The physicians concluded that the form was easy to use and that it also shortened the length of the patient visit. As a result of this small-scale test, primary care physicians at the TMC readily accepted use of the new documentation form in the initial months of the demonstration.

The sites approached initial implementation of the guideline differently depending on the gaps in practice and barriers to change they had identified at the kickoff conference. The sites initially emphasized different aspects of the guideline and different patient populations, although they all did so with the intent of eventually expanding these actions across the MTF. In all cases, however, the sites encountered difficulties in implementing the actions they had planned, and thus they had not undertaken the planned expansions as of the time of our second site visits.

Demonstration Site A. This site emphasized patient education and self-care, with the long-term goals of preventing recurrence of low back pain episodes and reducing the need for referrals to specialists. The site increased the capacity for the clinics and TMCs to offer back classes, and it established a formal process for specialty referrals, via a consult in the CHCS (the MTF's clinical information system). Referrals to back classes (patient education) were not monitored consistently, although staff reported an increase in such referrals. Compliance with the other components of the guideline was left to the discretion of the individual primary care providers working in the various clinics and TMCs.

Demonstration Site B. This site's primary goal for care of low back pain patients was to improve the timeliness of Medical Evaluation Board (MEB) assessments for active duty personnel with chronic low back pain. Consequently, the implementation team decided to introduce the guideline only in its TMCs, where those personnel are served. Adherence to the guideline was made optional at the family practice clinic, and the internal medicine clinic and the emergency room chose not to use it. This strategy was maintained throughout the demonstration. The site originally intended to integrate the guideline with a planned primary prevention effort using injury surveillance. Turnover in key staff, however, prevented implementation of this plan.

During the demonstration period, the number of low back pain encounters for active duty personnel increased by about 40 percent. Suggested reasons for the increase included improved tracking of visits and a change in practice requiring all active duty patients with low back pain to be seen by a PA. The number of referrals for MEB remained constant in 1999 but increased in the early part of 2000. Staff speculated that a forthcoming deployment to Bosnia may have accounted for this increase.

Demonstration Site C. This was the only site that took a comprehensive approach to implementing the low back pain guideline. The site sought to implement all components of the guidelines in all of its clinics and TMCs at the same time, and it used the low back pain documentation form 695-R as the primary vehicle to achieve the practices specified in the guideline. To overcome concerns by primary care providers that use of the form might increase patient processing time, the site had two TMC physicians test use of the form for one month. They concluded that the form not only was easy to use but also allowed for faster processing of patients. Use of the form was also extended to the occupational health clinic. The site intended to use selected metrics to assess progress and provide feedback to providers on potential issues or needed improvements, although this metrics capability was not fully implemented.

Compliance with use of form 695-R grew gradually during the early months of the demonstration but remained quite low (at about 20 percent). There was resistance to the form by nurses in the clinics who claimed they were too busy to add this extra burden to their workload. We do not know whether or how use of the form changed later in the demonstration because monitoring was discontinued due to staff time constraints, changes in MTF leadership, and turnover of the staff leading the implementation team.

Demonstration Site D. The initial primary concern of Site D was inappropriate referrals of low back pain patients to specialty care and a severe backlog of patients at the neurosurgery clinic. To address these issues, the site's physical medicine and rehabilitation clinic agreed to serve as a specialty resource for primary care providers and as a "gatekeeper" to assess and coordinate all specialty referrals of chronic low back pain patients. The primary care providers at the TMCs and hospital clinics were instructed to provide conservative treatment of low back pain patients during the first four to six weeks, after which patients were to be referred to the physical medicine clinic for assessment and appropriate follow-up treatment. The physical medicine clinic held weekly meetings with the relevant specialty care providers to coordinate the treatment of chronic low back pain patients referred by primary care providers.

On the acute low back pain side, primary care providers and physical therapists at Site D focused on standardizing their approach to conservative treatment, with specific attention to patient referrals to physical therapy. The occupational medicine clinic also began to use the guideline, and providers found it helped them manage care for low back pain patients. They also planned to introduce the guideline at the emergency department, which was staffed by contract physicians. These providers resisted use of the guideline, however, and the emergency department still had not yet begun to work with it as of the end of the demonstration. The primary care providers resisted use of the low back pain documentation form, so the site decided to postpone use of the form pending development of an electronic version of the guideline and of the form. It took nearly six months to complete the electronic form and integrate it into the site's clinical care software. The site began testing the new electronic form at one TMC a year after it began working with the low back pain guideline.

Trends in low back pain encounters reported by the site indicated that establishment of the gatekeeper function for chronic low back pain patients shifted encounters from the TMCs to the physical medicine clinic and reduced encounters in orthopedics and neurosurgery. The backlog of referrals to neurosurgery was cleared successfully. Total encounters remained relatively constant. These data did not make the distinction between patients referred during the six-week period of acute low back pain and those referred after they were considered to have chronic low back pain.

The Implementation Process and Activities

To carry out their respective strategies, the sites (1) introduced the guideline algorithm and supporting toolkit items to providers and staff, (2) sought to make changes to administrative procedures, (3) identified one standardized diagnostic code for low back pain, (4) provided patient education and self-management, and (5) monitored selected indicators. We synthesize the experiences of the four sites in each of these implementation steps and discuss the various approaches and activities they undertook.

Guideline Introduction and Training. All the sites began their implementation activities by holding education sessions for primary care providers to introduce them to the evidence-based practices specified in the low back pain guideline. The larger sites held separate sessions in each clinic. These initial sessions typically reached approximately 60 percent of the relevant providers, with absences reported to be due to deployments and work schedule conflicts. MEDCOM was securing CME credits for training on DoD/VA clinical guidelines but had not completed that process at the time of the initial education sessions. Some sites indicated that the absence of CME credit hindered participation in the training sessions. MEDCOM eventually got CME approval later in the demonstration period.

One site reported that contract and resource staff had incentives that discourage participation in training. Contractually, these providers are paid by the quantity of services they provide, and time spent in training diverts them from this activity.

The length of the training sessions ranged from less than an hour to half-day sessions, depending on the site. Providers attending the training sessions were given a copy of the practice guideline algorithms, and they discussed the purpose of the guideline, saw portions of the MEDCOM provider training video, and had an opportunity to ask questions and express their concerns. All sites reported that providers raised concerns about potential loss of autonomy (guidelines as "cookbook medicine") and about the additional visit time that might be required to use form 695-R. Of the providers who participated in focus groups during our site visits, an average of 75 percent reported they received a copy of the guideline, with a range across the sites of 40 to 100 percent. The site with the lowest percentage reported that it had experienced high turnover in clinical staff during the demonstration. About two-thirds of the providers participating in our focus groups rated the training sessions to be "very to extremely useful."

All sites recognized the need to offer additional training sessions for existing staff and newcomers, but only two of the sites actually carried out the additional training. One site provided additional education for providers at two of its clinics by spending 20 minutes on the low back pain guideline within the context of a three-hour education session that focused primarily on the asthma and diabetes guidelines. Another site, having experienced turnover of one-half of its staff during the demonstration, integrated an introduction to the low back pain guideline into its two-day orientation to the hospital for newcomers.

None of the sites held formal training sessions for nurses, medics, PAs, or other ancillary staff involved in the treatment of low back pain patients. In most cases, these staff were simply instructed to ask patients to fill out their portion of form 695-R and, at some sites, to hand out a patient education pamphlet. Only about one-half of the ancillary staff that participated in our focus groups reported they had been introduced to the guideline. This omission contributed to reluctance by clinic staff at some sites to cooperate in using the guideline.

Procedures to Document Care. To ensure use of conservative treatment for acute low back pain patients, all sites attempted to use the encounter form 695-R to support implementation of the guideline and ensure documentation of diagnosis and treatment. Compliance varied across the sites, however, depending on the support availability and frequency of rotation of ancillary staff, acceptance of the form by primary care providers, and aggressiveness of monitoring.

Typically, a low back pain patient was identified at the sign-in desk or in the screening room. The patient was asked to fill out the patient portion of the form. Clinic staff filled in the vital signs section and attached the form to the medical chart for the provider's use. Compliance with this relatively simple procedure varied initially from 20 percent at some clinics to 92 percent at some TMCs, and most sites reported that compliance decreased over time.

Several reasons were given for low compliance with use of the documentation form. First, it was not clear to the sites whether MEDCOM mandated use of the form or gave the sites the discretion to decide whether and how to use it. MEDCOM clarified that the sites were expected to document the diagnosis and treatment of low back pain patients appropriately in the medical chart, but they could choose how to do that. The form 695-R was provided as a tool that would achieve appropriate documentation, but they were not required to use it. In response to this guidance, the sites tended to leave to the individual providers the decision about whether to use form 695-R.

A second reason for low compliance in using form 695-R is that many providers were not satisfied with the contents of the form, and in particular, many complained that the form did not provide enough space to write notes. Overall, most physicians reported they used the form at the first visit (65 percent of providers in the focus groups), but only 20 percent used it at subsequent visits or for patients presenting with multiple problems. Providers felt that filling out the form at each return visit was duplicative and unnecessary. At one site, physicians had all but stopped using the form by the time of our last visit. Lack of standardization among providers within one clinic or TMC in use of the form made the processing of patients confusing for the ancillary staff.

Third, many ancillary staff perceived that the documentation form added to an already heavy workload, and, hence, they were reluctant to use it. Ironically, about two-thirds of the ancillary staff that participated in our focus groups and had used the form reported that it shortened processing time (45 percent) or made no difference

(22 percent). Some providers reported they did not insist the form be included with the patient's chart because they knew the ancillary staff were overworked and they did not like placing new demands on them.

The relatively high rotation of ancillary staff, particularly at TMCs, also contributed to low compliance with use of form 695-R. The sites did not act forcefully to maintain adequate levels of staff training regarding procedures for use of the form. Finally, some TMCs and clinics reported they ran out of forms and did not know how to replace them. MEDCOM did not set down procedures for ordering new supplies until later in the demonstration. This administrative barrier for providers and clinic staff discouraged use of the form yet further.

The sites encountered other issues in working with form 695-R. For example, one issue involved the placement of the form in the chart. AMEDD regulations state that only the SF-600 form can be placed in chronological order in the patient chart. All other forms must be placed at the end or on the left side. Providers at some sites expressed frustration at having to search for the form in the chart.

Seeking to overcome some of these difficulties, one site spent considerable staff time to develop an automated form 695-R. The use of this automated form was being tested at one TMC at the time of our last visit, but test results were not yet available.

Standardization of ADS Reporting. To facilitate monitoring of how use of the guideline affected low back pain care, MEDCOM worked with the demonstration sites to identify one diagnostic code for low back pain (724.2) that all MTFs should use to code low back pain visits. In addition, coding was added to the MTF section of the ADS sheet to distinguish between acute and chronic cases. As of the end of the demonstration period, the sites were still not using the designated low back pain diagnostic code, continuing instead to use multiple codes to record low back pain visits. One site, however, added an indicator to the ADS form for acute versus chronic low back pain, and another site added an indicator for attending back class.

Patient Education. Patient education was at the core of the guideline implementation strategy at one site. Its physical therapy clinic developed a one-hour back class curriculum that covered common causes of back pain and injuries, body mechanics, and stretching and strengthening exercises. Medics or nurses led the classes. This site increased access to back classes by offering them at each of its hospital clinics and TMCs and by increasing the total number of available classes. Classes were held either weekly or twice a month, depending on demand. Providers were asked to refer all first-time low back pain patients to back classes. At some TMCs, staff secured the cooperation of unit commanders to allow soldiers to attend the back classes. Even with these improvements, however, patient no-show rates were high. The site did not have a system to follow up with patients who did not attend the classes to encourage future attendance. The form used was simply stamped "no-show."

Another site also encouraged patients to attend back classes, but referrals were at the discretion of the provider. Similar to the previous site, this site made referrals and did not follow up with no-show patients.

The other two sites made no procedural changes in the way they referred low back pain patients to back classes. It was left to the providers' discretion to tell patients about the availability of back classes. One of these sites offered back classes at its wellness center, to which providers referred retirees and family members but did not refer active duty personnel. The other site had a wellness center, but providers did not refer low back pain patients to it. Patients might be given a copy of the patient education pamphlet, but the provider was the main source of patient education.

Two of the sites showed the patient education video in waiting rooms in addition to showing it in back classes. The sites that did not show the video cited barriers in the physical layout of waiting rooms and lack of video equipment as reasons for not doing so.

Monitoring and Feedback. Although the sites were encouraged to use various metrics to monitor implementation progress, they were slow to do so. One reason was that the expert panel for the DoD/VA guideline did not finalize its list of recommended metrics until several months after the demonstration kickoff conference. The sites eventually selected some indicators to track, with each site identifying a different set of indicators. One site made extensive use of the ADS and CHCS data to track trends in low back pain encounters and dispositions. The other sites limited their tracking to the number of encounters. Staff at the sites had some difficulty retrieving ADS and CHCS data because they were not accustomed to using the system for monitoring and management purposes. The MTFs varied substantially in the availability of personnel with the programming ability to extract data from the CHCS.

Three sites used chart reviews to monitor the presence of the documentation form 695-R in the chart and documentation of the red-flag conditions. With one exception, the sites completed only one round of chart reviews, so they were not able to track trends. The sites were reluctant to undertake chart reviews on a regular basis because they are time consuming to perform. Staff also had a tendency to do one review with a large sample of charts rather than performing a series of reviews of smaller samples each. Difficulty in locating medical charts added significantly to the chart review time demands. For example, 300 patients were sampled at one site, for whom 60 charts could be located and only 27 were actually reviewed.

The chart reviews revealed large variations in the presence of form 695-R in the charts across sites and also across TMCs and clinics within sites. Completeness ranged from 100 percent at one TMC to 20 percent or less at some clinics. Compliance with use of the form was typically higher at TMCs than clinics. The two sites that extracted information on the documentation of red-flag conditions found low rates of compliance (19 percent and 15 percent, respectively).

A majority of providers participating in the focus groups indicated they had seen some monitoring data on their treatment of low back pain patients during the demonstration. However, none of the sites reported having used the monitoring data to undertake corrective actions.

LESSONS LEARNED

Although the MTFs participating in the low back pain guideline demonstration had some notable successes in some aspects of improving low back pain treatment practices, the overall progress made during the demonstration was quite limited. Of particular concern was the inability of the MTFs to sustain early achievements in introducing new practices. Important contributing factors to this result were the generally tepid support from the MTF command teams, which was compounded by turnover of key personnel leading the implementation activities. We summarize here some of the specific lessons learned from this demonstration, which generated rich information that has been used by MEDCOM for subsequent demonstrations as well as for introduction of the low back pain practice guideline across all Army treatment facilities.

Flexibility Versus Consistency

The MTFs used the flexibility they were given to establish a variety of implementation strategies, which reflected each MTF's unique capabilities and circumstances. The MTFs emphasized different components of the guideline, and they differed in how broadly they implemented it across their clinics and TMCs. Although we believe this flexibility helps to ensure that each MTF can address the clinic practices most in need of improvement, it also may slow progress toward the AMEDD goal of achieving consistent practices across its facilities. Documentation of variations in key practices across MTFs, such as we presented in Chapter Three, should be performed routinely to identify areas where improvements in quality and consistency are needed. With this information in hand, MEDCOM can determine whether to give the MTFs greater direction regarding which aspects of the guideline are to be implemented uniformly.

Monitoring and Accountability

Monitoring of progress in changing practices became almost an afterthought in this demonstration, as a result of the newness of the AMEDD practice guideline initiative. The low back pain demonstration was the first demonstration, the official low back pain guideline metrics were late to be completed, and MEDCOM did not have the resources or time to establish a monitoring system and related data. The absence of monitoring weakened accountability for the MTFs, but accountability would have stimulated their continued efforts to achieve the desired new practices. Thus this absence contributed to limited progress in affecting treatment processes for low back pain patients.

Coding and Data Retrieval

Several measurement issues arose during the demonstration that hampered effective monitoring, specifically inconsistencies in coding low back pain visits and challenges in retrieving ADS and CHCS data for use in the monitoring process. Accurate coding of low back pain visits in the ADS data is required to identify these patients for analysis. In collaboration with the sites, MEDCOM established a standard low back pain diagnostic code, but the sites did not consistently use this code, reportedly because of staff time constraints. MTF staff also had difficulty retrieving CHCS data and ADS data, and special "ad hoc" programs were needed to extract CHCS data. MEDCOM will need to provide instructions and ongoing support to help MTFs overcome these issues as well as others that may be compromising the ability to do effective monitoring.

Ongoing Provider/Staff Education

At the start of the demonstration, the participating MTFs generally provided effective education for providers on the low back pain practice guideline. However, it quickly became apparent that it would be a challenge to achieve high levels of knowledge of the guideline contents for providers and to maintain knowledge levels as providers rotated in and out of the MTFs over time. In addition, the sites did not educate other clinic staff on the new guideline, which hampered the ability of some sites to implement new procedures involving those staff. To ensure knowledge and buy-in over time, MTFs will need to provide ongoing education for existing personnel and include guideline information in the orientation sessions for incoming staff.

Patient Education

According to the low back pain practice guideline, patients should play an active role in managing their back pain through self-care, exercises, and lifestyle modifications. Although all the sites undertook some patient education, and some increased the use of patient back classes, only one site made patient education an important part of its strategy. All sites reported difficulty in motivating patients to assume responsibility for part of their care. This issue of the need for and difficulty of patient education will apply to many of the practice guidelines AMEDD will implement, most of which are for chronic conditions. MEDCOM could assist its MTFs by further defining the role of patient education and self-care support in treatment processes and by providing them tested educational methods and resources.

Defining New Procedures and Responsibility for Them

The demonstration highlighted the importance of establishing clear procedures for new clinical processes being introduced by an MTF. Uncertainty about any of the specific steps of a new procedure discourages providers and clinic staff from adopting it and thus becomes a barrier to implementing new practices. In some cases, such as regulations regarding placement of a documentation form in a medical chart, MEDCOM has the responsibility to revise procedures to support use of new practices. In other cases, such as specifying clearly which staff are responsible for completing the encounter documentation form, the responsibility belongs to the MTFs.

Integrating New Practices

Perhaps the most important lesson from the low back pain demonstration was the importance—and difficulty—of successfully integrating new practices into the way MTFs routinely "do business" for patient care. A practice guideline can be said to be implemented only when such lasting changes in practices are made. Few of the MTFs participating in the demonstration were able to maintain the new practices they introduced at the start of the implementation period. A variety of reasons for this inability to "institutionalize" the new practices can be identified, depending on the site and practice involved, including limited leadership support, inadequate buy-in from providers or clinic staff, lack of clarity of roles and responsibilities, and absence of monitoring and feedback on progress. As guidelines are introduced across the AMEDD system, ongoing monitoring and technical support from MEDCOM will be needed to help ensure the retention of desired new practices for treatment of patients served by the Army MTFs.

Chapter Six

EFFECTS OF GUIDELINE IMPLEMENTATION

In this chapter, we examine the extent to which introduction of the low back pain guideline at the four demonstration MTFs changed clinical practices in those facilities. Using information from the process evaluation and the analysis of encounter data, we (1) assessed how well providers at the demonstration sites appeared to understand and accept the guideline, (2) summarized reports from the sites regarding estimates from their analyses of the effects of their implementation activities on clinical practices, and (3) analyzed trends of service utilization for the six identified indicators of low back pain care, comparing the demonstration sites with control sites that had not used the guideline. We synthesize the results of these three analyses to identify areas where demonstration site practices appeared to change and where the perceptions of the sites differed from results of the independent data analysis.

PROVIDER KNOWLEDGE AND ACCEPTANCE OF THE GUIDELINE

Provider Knowledge and Views of the Low Back Pain Guideline

Primary care providers participating in the RAND site visits generally acknowledged the guideline was a potentially useful resource, but many of them viewed it without much enthusiasm. Acceptance varied widely across demonstration sites and among primary care providers within each site. Nurse practitioners and PAs had more favorable views of the guideline than physicians because it offered them potential for greater autonomy and technical support as they treated low back pain patients, reducing their need to turn frequently to providers for guidance. Providers expressed a range of positive and negative views about the guideline. For example, we heard statements that the guideline

- "stimulates an emphasis on prevention and patient self-management"
- "provides specific guidance for when to refer a patient for more definitive diagnostic procedures"
- "helps reduce referrals to physical therapy and specialists"
- "should increase the quality, continuity, and consistency of care"
- "will have no impact on care . . . because we are already following the guideline"
- "will increase workload for documentation and staff time spent in meetings."

At the end of the demonstration, we asked providers participating in our focus groups their views about clinical practice guidelines in general and the low back pain guideline in particular. In excess of 90 percent of providers agreed "slightly" to "strongly" with the statements that clinical practice guidelines help deliver better care, reduce variations in clinical practice, and are a good way to summarize and reenforce scientific evidence on diagnosis and management of specific conditions. At the same time, a significant minority (from 20 to 35 percent) thought that clinical practice guidelines oversimplify diagnostic and treatment decisions in medicine, limit a physician's freedom to take action, and reduce provider efficiency. When asked about the low back pain guideline, none of the providers agreed with the statements that the low back pain guideline "has reduced my flexibility to treat low back pain patients" or "has increased the time I spend with low back pain patients." These results suggest that providers have mixed attitudes toward clinical practice guidelines in general, which could become more positive over time as the providers gain more hands-on experience working with guidelines for specific conditions.

By the end of the demonstration, many providers were knowledgeable about the conservative treatment recommended by the guideline for acute low back pain patients, but a sizable minority still had not gained that knowledge. For instance, 25 percent of the providers responding to our survey did not know or remember that the guideline prescribes no more than 48 hours of bed rest, and one in three providers did not know the guideline does not recommend the use of muscle relaxants for management of pain. At one site, 60 percent of the providers surveyed did not know these guideline provisions.

Effects of the Guideline on Providers' Behavior

A majority of the providers participating in our focus groups reported the guideline had improved the way they deliver care for low back pain patients. Of those responding to our survey, 60 percent agreed with the statement that "the guideline had helped me to provide better care for my low back pain patients" and with the statement that "the guideline has reduced variations in the way I treat low back pain patients." These proportions varied across sites from 100 percent of providers at one site to a low of 40 percent at another. Providers also generally agreed that the guideline had not "increased the time I spent with low back pain patients."

Only about one-half the providers agreed with the statement on the survey that the guideline "is applicable to all low back pain patients" because many of them believed the guideline was not applicable to military basic trainees: These trainees stay on post for only a short period of time, and when a trainee has a health problem, the MTF is under heavy pressure to return her or him to duty as rapidly as possible to minimize interruption of training. Providers reported that the key question they ask themselves for one of these patients is, "If I let this individual return to basic training while the back pain is still present, will the training harm her or him?"

REPORTED CHANGES IN CLINICAL PRACTICES

Implementation of the low back pain guideline led three of the four sites to make changes in clinical practices, some of which may have been maintained successfully as routine practices. To examine this question, we asked the implementation team and providers in our focus group which practice changes they think occurred and any evidence they had that documented such changes. We also obtained reports from some sites with data they had developed on trends of low back pain encounters.

Primary Care Services

Three of the demonstration sites analyzed data on frequency of encounters and length of treatment, the results of which suggested there was general adherence with conservative treatment of low back pain patients, as recommended by the guideline. One site reported that 47 percent of patients had only one encounter for low back pain. Another reported that two-thirds of its low back pain patients had no more than two encounters and another 20 percent of its patients had three encounters. Both sites reported that less than 2 percent of low back pain patients had seven or more encounters. A small number of patients had an unusually large number of low back pain encounters, and these patients were identified for follow-up and potential reassessment.

At the site that began to require all new low back pain patients to attend back class before they could be referred to physical therapy or specialty care, back class attendance increased, but there still were high no-show rates at the classes. This site also changed its practice in the emergency room, asking ER staff to triage patients presenting with low back pain for red-flag conditions, treat those with serious problems, and send the remaining patients directly to their primary care provider for conservative treatment. In the past, the ER staff would attempt to manage low back pain patients on a continuing basis. This change in procedure might result in an increase in observed follow-up visits.

One site reported that 56 percent of its low back pain patients were in care for one month or less and another 16 percent between one and two months. Less than 10 percent of patients were in care for six months or more.

Change in Patterns of Referrals

Primary care providers said they changed their patterns of specialty referrals to be more consistent with conservative treatment of acute back pain patients. Providers responding to our survey at the second site visits were asked: "Has the low back pain guideline led *you* to increase or decrease your referrals to the following services?" Overall, they reported that referrals to back classes, physical therapy, chiropractors (where available), and dieticians increased, but that referrals to X ray, CT scan, MRI, neurosurgery, and orthopedics decreased or remained the same. In contrast with the primary care provider reports, neurosurgery and orthopedics specialists at the demonstration sites indicated that they continued to receive inappropriate referrals that represented an estimated 10 to 30 percent of the total patients referred to them.

In interpreting these reports, the reader should keep two limitations in mind. First, the reported changes reflect the providers' perceptions of changes in their behavior, which may have differed from actual changes as measured with encounter data. Second, the providers who participated in the focus groups probably were not representative of all providers at the MTFs. These providers (some of whom were members of the implementation teams) were likely to be more knowledgeable about the guideline than others who did not participate in the focus groups, and they were also likely to be readier to adopt new practices stated in the guideline.

One site changed its handling of chronic low back pain cases. The primary care clinics began to refer all persistent cases to the physical medicine clinic for assessment by a multidisciplinary team and referral to the appropriate specialist(s) and, if necessary, to permanent profiling or the MEB. Treatment of difficult cases was coordinated in weekly meetings of a multidisciplinary team. According to the site, this practice eliminated a chronic backlog of neurosurgery referrals and helped to standardize the treatment of chronic low back pain patients.

Change in Prescription of Pharmaceuticals

Providers perceived that prescriptions of pharmaceuticals had changed in a manner consistent with the guideline recommendations. They reported they had shifted to prescribing NSAIDs more frequently for initial pain management, rather than narcotics, and also to prescribing another NSAID if the patient does not adequately respond to the first NSAID. However, they also reported that they continued to prescribe muscle relaxants, with little or no change from previous practices.

Staff Perceptions of Patient Satisfaction

The majority of providers and ancillary staff perceived that the guideline had no effect on satisfaction and self-care for low back pain patients. We asked providers and ancillary staff about their level of agreement or disagreement with five statements about patient satisfaction, responsibility for care, and health behaviors. Overall, less than one-third of the respondents agreed that low back pain patients were more satisfied with the care received, took more responsibility for self-care, and were returning to duty earlier than they otherwise would have. A similar proportion agreed with the statement that low back pain patients complained more often that they had not received the treatment they expected, which was an anticipated patient response to any reduction in interventions involved in conservative treatment. The same limitations identified above apply to interpreting these responses to these survey items.

Provider and clinic staff opinions about the effects of the guideline on patients varied across the demonstration sites, in part reflecting their respective levels of acceptance and use of the guideline. Providers' opinions about effects on patients also differed somewhat from those of the ancillary staff, although we found no overall pattern to those differences.

ANALYSIS OF EFFECTS ON CLINICAL PRACTICES

The results of the analysis of trends in clinical practices for low back pain patients are reported here. We compare the practices of the demonstration sites before and after they started working with the low back pain practice guideline, and also with the practices of five control sites that were not part of the demonstration. Refer to Chapter Two and Appendix A for details on the methods used for this analysis.

The Study Population

The analysis was based on episodes of care for acute low back pain. Each episode was defined to start with an initial visit for low back pain that was not preceded by a similar visit during the previous 90 days. Utilization data for five quarter-years were included in the study, two quarters before the demonstration MTFs began implementing the low back pain guideline and three quarters during the demonstration period. Each episode of care was assigned to the quarter-year in which the initial visit for that episode occurred. Then for each episode of care in the study sample, we extracted all subsequent MTF outpatient encounters and MTF pharmacy records for a six-month period following the date of the initial visit.

There were a total of 31,273 initial encounters for new episodes of low back pain in the analysis, roughly one-half of which occurred in the demonstration MTFs and one-half in the control MTFs, as shown in Table 6.1. The number of encounters remained relatively stable over time, as shown in Table 6.2. Of the initial low back pain encounters, 83 percent occurred in primary care–type clinics, including primary care (41 percent), family practice (37 percent), internal medicine (one percent), and flight medicine (three percent). Eight

Table 6.1

Number and Percentage of New Low Back Pain Patient Encounters

	New Low Back Pain Patients	
MTF Group	Number	Percentage
Demonstration sites	16,299	52.1
Site A	7,112	22.7
Site B	2,460	7.9
Site C	4,039	12.9
Site D	2,688	8.6
Great Plains control sites	5,082	16.3
Site C1	1,445	4.6
Site C2	1,992	6.4
Site C3	1,645	5.3
Other control sites	9,892	31.6
Site C4	3,383	10.8
Site C5	6,509	20.8
Total	31,273	100.0

Table 6.2

New Low Back Pain Patient Encounters, by Site and Quarter

MTF Groups	1st Qtr, 1999	2nd Qtr, 1999	3rd Qtr, 1999	4th Qtr, 1999	1st Qtr, 2000
Demonstration sites	3,159	3,576	3,095	3,508	2,961
Great Plains control sites	989	1,029	1,063	986	1,015
Other control sites	1,896	2,043	1,957	2,062	1,934

percent occurred in emergency rooms, five percent occurred in orthopedic clinics, and four percent occurred in other settings.

Measures and Methods

As described in Chapter Two, six indicators were selected for analysis in the evaluation. All the indicators address aspects of care for acute low back pain patients (i.e., during the first six weeks of care following the initial low back pain visit). In Chapter Three, we presented the baseline performance of all the demonstration and control MTFs on these indicators. In this chapter, we examine the extent to which the indicators changed for the demonstration sites during the period they implemented new practices for the low back pain guideline. These indicators address the following aspects of care in the first six weeks after an initial low back pain visit:

1. percentage of patients referred to physical therapy or manipulation
2. number of follow-up visits per patient for low back pain patients
3. percentage of acute low back pain patients referred to specialty care
4. percentage of acute low back pain patients prescribed muscle relaxants
5. percentage of acute low back pain patients prescribed narcotics
6. percentage of NSAIDs prescribed that are high cost.

Expected reductions in these indicators are based on the assumption that an MTF effectively introduces and maintains the new approach of conservative treatment. Therefore, we would expect to observe hypothesized changes in clinical practices only in those MTFs that proactively worked to implement the new practices. In addition, we also expect that the particular intervention strategy of each MTF will determine which effects will be observed in the analysis. For example, there should be a reduction in referrals to specialty care only for those MTFs that defined specialty referrals as a priority and actually undertook actions to reduce inappropriate referrals.

For each of the six indicators, we present the average values by quarter for the demonstration sites and for each of the two groups of control sites, and we provide graphs showing trends visually. We collapsed the two control groups for all the trend analyses and tests of significance because there the trends for the two groups did not differ for any of the measures. To test the significance of observed trends for each metric, we fit a multivariate regression model with predictor variables for demonstration versus control, individual facility, and quarter. Interaction terms were used to test differences in rates during the demonstration period relative to the two baseline quarters. We controlled for patient gender, age, and rank in these models. Appendix C presents the detailed results of the multivariate modeling.

Referrals to Physical Therapy or Manipulation

We hypothesized that use of the guideline would lead to reductions in physical therapy and manipulation services as MTFs increasingly used the conservative treatment approach. To test this hypothesis, we examined trends in the percentage of acute low back pain patients referred to these services within six weeks of the initial low back pain encounter. A total of 3,181 patients were referred for physical therapy or manipulation services across the five quarters, about one-half of them in the demonstration MTFs and one-half in the control MTFs (Table 6.3). After introducing the guideline, physical therapy referral rates declined at the demonstration sites but did not decline at the control sites. In the second quarter of 1999, 11 percent of low back pain patients at the demonstration sites were referred to physical therapy or manipulation services (Table 6.3 and

Table 6.3

Patients Referred to Physical Therapy or Manipulation Within Six Weeks of Initial Low Back Pain Encounter, by MTF and Quarter

	Number of	Percentage Referred				
MTF Groups	Patients Referred	1st Qtr, 1999	2nd Qtr, 1999	3rd Qtr, 1999	4th Qtr, 1999	1st Qtr, 2000
Demonstration sites	1,476	10.0	10.7	9.5	7.8	7.2
Site A	494	6.9	9.7	9.6	4.6	4.0
Site B	298	11.5	14.0	9.6	12.1	13.1
Site C	448	16.5	10.5	8.8	9.1	10.3
Site D	236	6.7	10.0	9.8	11.4	4.9
Great Plains control sites	683	13.4	16.8	11.8	11.9	13.3
Site C1	203	14.6	18.9	8.5	15.4	13.8
Site C2	222	10.9	12.5	11.3	7.7	13.0
Site C3	258	15.5	20.7	15.4	13.5	13.2
Other control sites	1,022	8.4	11.1	10.2	11.5	10.3
Site C4	319	8.9	10.9	8.4	9.7	9.3
Site C5	703	8.2	11.2	11.2	12.5	10.8

Figure 6.1). By the first quarter of 2000, only 7 percent were referred. This trend was statistically significant for quarters 4 and 5 (see Appendix C).

Site B was the only one showing no decline in physical therapy or manipulation referral rates, and this site had taken very little action in implementing the guideline. We did a separate graph of the trend in rates for the other three demonstration sites, excluding Site B, to assess the strength of effect for the MTFs that did take actions in this area. The downward trend in referral rates for the remaining three demonstration sites became more pronounced, as shown in the third trend line in Figure 6.1.

There was substantial variation across the demonstration sites in physical therapy referral trends (see Figure 6.2). This variation is consistent with observations of the implementation process at the demonstration sites. Site A had made the strongest reduction in physical therapy referrals, and Site C made a moderate early reduction in referrals that remained stable in subsequent quarters. Site D had a reduction in the last quarter, and Site B had no effect at all on physical therapy or manipulation referrals.

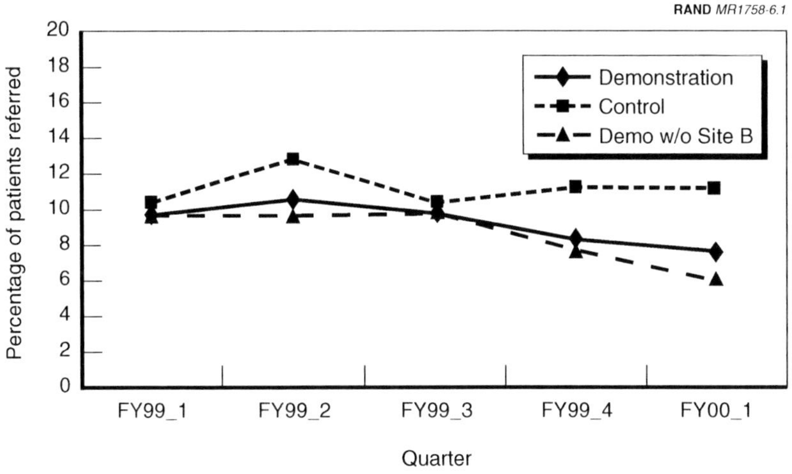

Figure 6.1—Trends in Percentage of Acute Low Back Pain Patients Referred for Physical Therapy or Manipulation Care, Demonstration and Control Sites

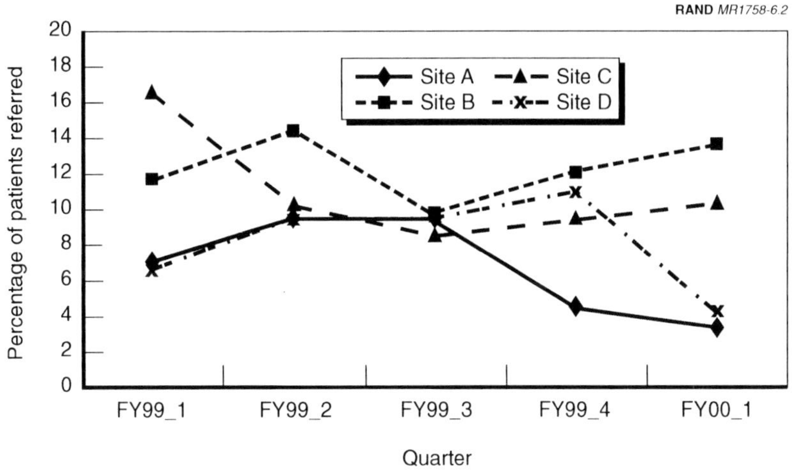

Figure 6.2—Trends in Percentage of Acute Low Back Pain Patients Referred for Physical Therapy or Manipulation Care, Individual Demonstration Sites

Follow-Up Primary Care Visits

We hypothesized that the conservative treatment recommendations of the guideline would decrease the number of follow-up primary care visits for new low back pain patients because MTF providers would encourage more self-care. The 31,273 new low back pain patients had a total of 27,187 follow-up primary care visits within six weeks of the initial low back pain encounters. There was no discernible trend in the average number of follow-up visits for the demonstration sites, while the average number of visits per patient gradually increased at the control sites (Table 6.4 and Figure 6.3). The decline in follow-up visits per patient for the last quarter in the demonstration sites, compared with the control sites, was found to be statistically significant (see Appendix C). Looking at the individual demonstration sites, there was little variation across the sites in trends for average number of follow-up primary care visits (Figure 6.4).

Table 6.4

Average Number of Follow-Up Primary Care Visits Per Patient, by MTF and Quarter

MTF Groups	Number of New Patients	Average Number of Follow-Up Visits Per Person				
		1st Qtr, 1999	2nd Qtr, 1999	3rd Qtr, 1999	4th Qtr, 1999	1st Qtr, 2000
Demonstration sites	16,299	0.88	0.91	0.89	0.90	0.86
Site A	7,112	0.90	0.89	0.93	0.96	0.89
Site B	2,460	0.75	0.75	0.77	0.75	0.65
Site C	4,039	0.99	1.09	1.00	1.00	1.01
Site D	2,688	0.80	0.86	0.74	0.72	0.70
Great Plains control sites	5,082	0.79	0.76	0.75	0.79	0.83
Site C1	1,445	0.66	0.62	0.65	0.72	0.83
Site C2	1,992	0.92	0.90	0.89	0.90	0.91
Site C3	1,645	0.70	0.68	0.69	0.72	0.80
Other control sites	9,892	0.81	0.81	0.84	0.84	0.84
Site C4	3,383	0.71	0.70	0.80	0.74	0.74
Site C5	6,509	0.86	0.87	0.87	0.89	0.89

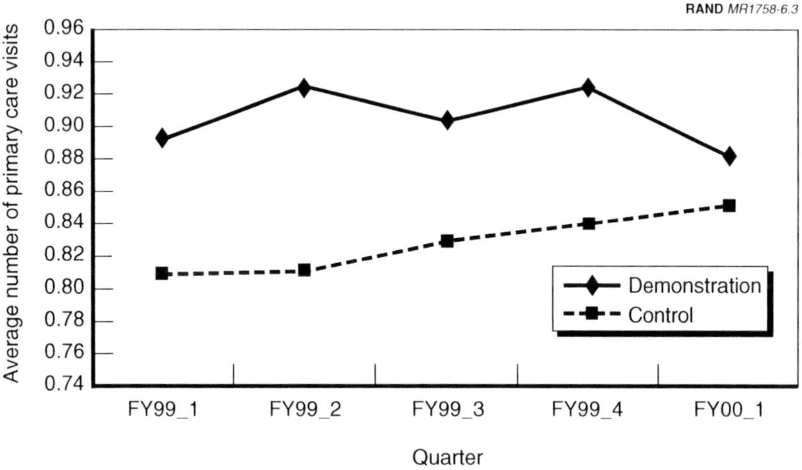

Figure 6.3—Trends in the Number of Follow-Up Primary Care Visits Per Patient for Acute Low Back Pain Patients, Demonstration and Control Sites

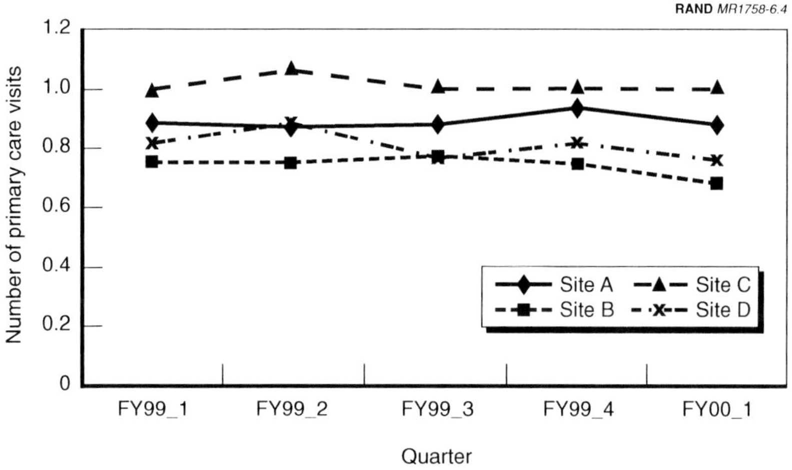

Figure 6.4—Trends in the Number of Follow-Up Primary Care Visits Per Patient for Acute Low Back Pain Patients, by Demonstration MTF

Referrals to Specialty Care

We hypothesized that use of the low back pain guideline would reduce referral rates to specialty providers for acute low back pain patients during the six weeks of conservative treatment. The specialties included in these analyses were orthopedics, neurology, neurosurgery, and physical medicine and rehabilitation. A total of 3,750 acute low back pain patients had a specialty care visit within six weeks of the initial low back pain visit (Table 6.5). Specialty referral patterns differed across the MTFs in terms of both rates and the types of specialties to which referrals were made. The majority of specialty referrals were to orthopedists, who saw an average of 56 percent of the specialty referrals at the demonstration sites and 48 percent of the referrals at the control sites (Figures 6.5 and 6.6). The second most common specialty referral was to physical medicine/rehabilitation. Two control MTFs and one demonstration MTF had no neurology referrals, and two other control sites and one other demonstration site had no neurosurgery referrals.

Table 6.5

Percentage of Patients Referred to Specialty Care Within Six Weeks of Initial Low Back Pain Encounter, by MTF and Quarter

MTF Group	Number of Patients Referred	Percentage Referred 1st Qtr, 1999	2nd Qtr, 1999	3rd Qtr, 1999	4th Qtr, 1999	1st Qtr, 2000
Demonstration sites	1,752	13.4	10.5	10.4	9.7	9.8
Site A	661	12.4	10.1	9.4	7.9	7.1
Site B	360	12.3	14.7	14.8	12.8	19.2
Site C	275	14.2	4.2	5.1	5.9	4.7
Site D	456	15.7	16.3	16.2	18.2	19.0
Great Plains control sites	759	15.6	16.7	15.6	14.9	11.8
Site C1	229	15.9	18.2	17.7	15.8	11.8
Site C2	157	8.7	10.2	7.8	6.6	5.7
Site C3	373	23.5	24.1	22.8	23.9	19.0
Other control sites	1,239	15.5	13.3	11.5	11.9	10.5
Site C4	586	19.4	18.5	15.3	18.2	15.2
Site C5	653	13.4	10.8	9.3	8.7	8.1

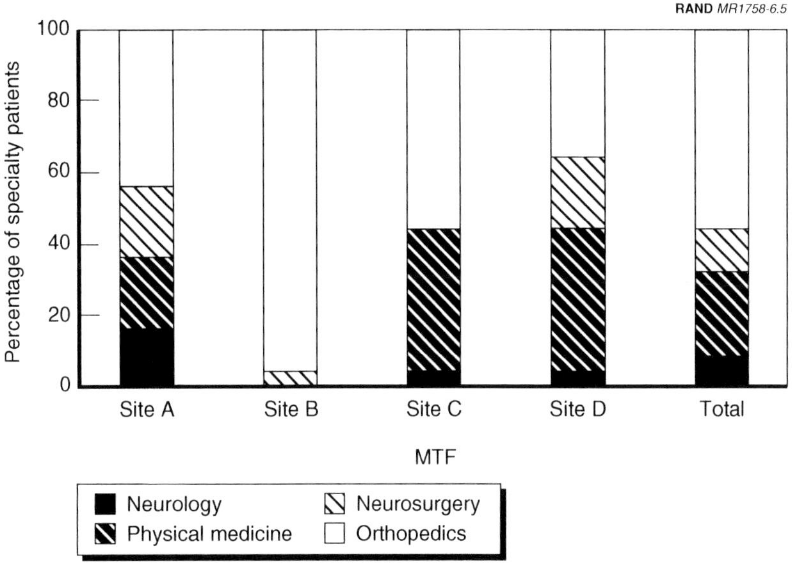

Figure 6.5—Distribution of Specialty Referrals for Acute Low Back Pain Patients by Type of Specialty, Demonstration MTFs

Overall, we found that introduction of the guideline did not appear to affect rates of specialty care referrals for acute low back pain patients. The percentage of patients referred to specialists was relatively stable at the demonstration MTFs over the last three quarters, while percentages declined over time at the control MTFs (Table 6.5 and Figure 6.7). However, underlying the overall lack of trend in the demonstration MTFs were slight declines in specialty referral rates at three MTFs, while referral rates to orthopedists increased markedly at one demonstration MTF during the last two quarters of the study period. When we checked with the MTF to identify possible reasons for this increase, staff were not able to identify any change in staffing or practice patterns that might explain it. We excluded this MTF from a second analysis to test its effect on overall trends, and we found that the remaining demonstration MTFs had a downward trend in specialty referrals similar to that for the control MTFs (Figure 6.8). Statistical tests (see Appendix C) showed that the trend for the three

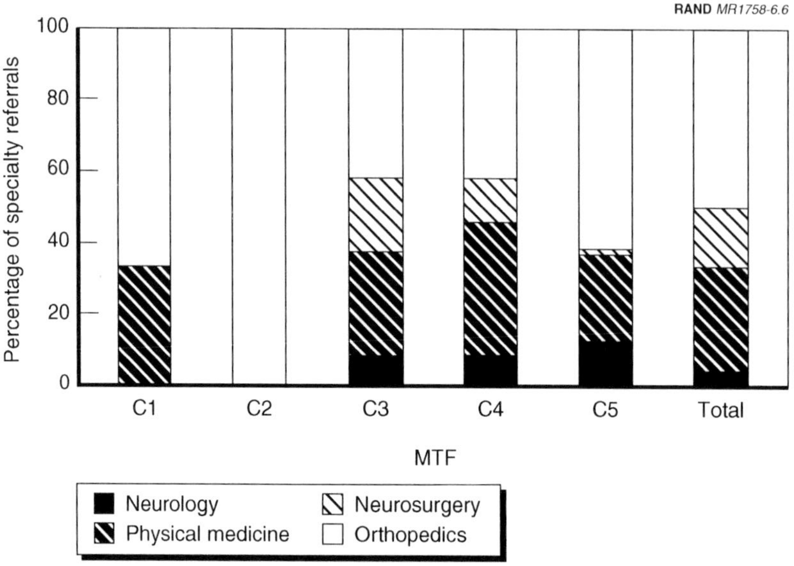

Figure 6.6—Distribution of Specialty Referrals for Acute Low Back Pain Patients by Type of Specialty, Control MTFs

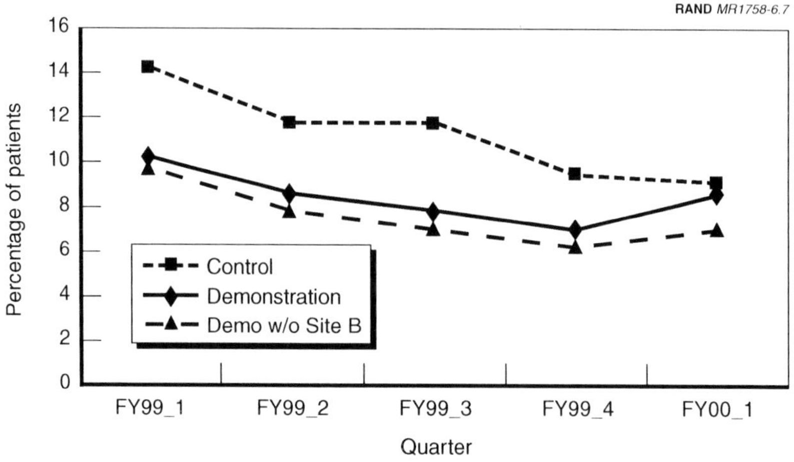

Figure 6.7—Trends in the Percentage of Acute Low Back Pain Patients Referred for Specialty Care, Demonstration and Control Sites

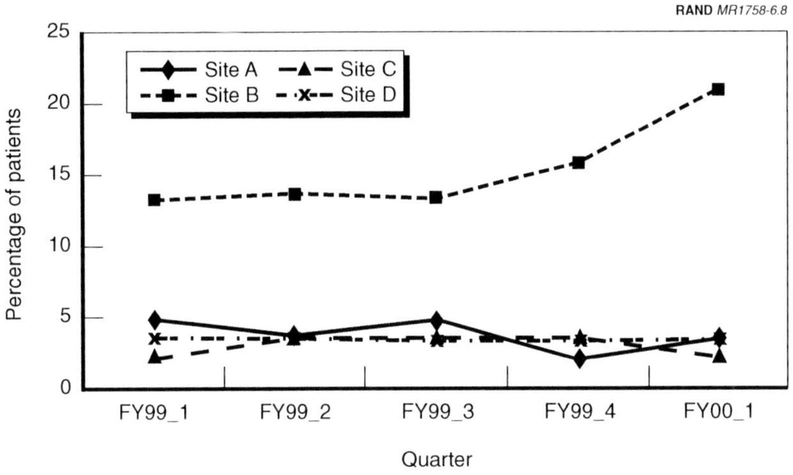

Figure 6.8—Trends in the Percentage of Acute Low Back Pain Patients Referred for Specialty Care, by Demonstration Site

demonstration sites (excluding Site B) was not significantly different from the trend for the control sites. In either model, we found no guideline effect on overall rates of specialty referrals.

Despite the absence of an overall guideline effect on specialty referrals, the trend in specialty mix at one demonstration site, Site D, represented successful implementation of a key element of its action plan. The site shifted low back pain referrals away from other specialties and toward physical medicine and rehabilitation, which took on the gatekeeper role for low back pain care (see Figure 6.9).

Prescription of Muscle Relaxants

The low back pain guideline specifically states that the scientific evidence shows that muscle relaxants do not help ease the back pain, and therefore they should not be prescribed for patients. Given that muscle relaxants were prescribed for almost one-half of the acute low back pain patients at the demonstration and control sites before the demonstration, as shown in Chapter Three, we hypothesized

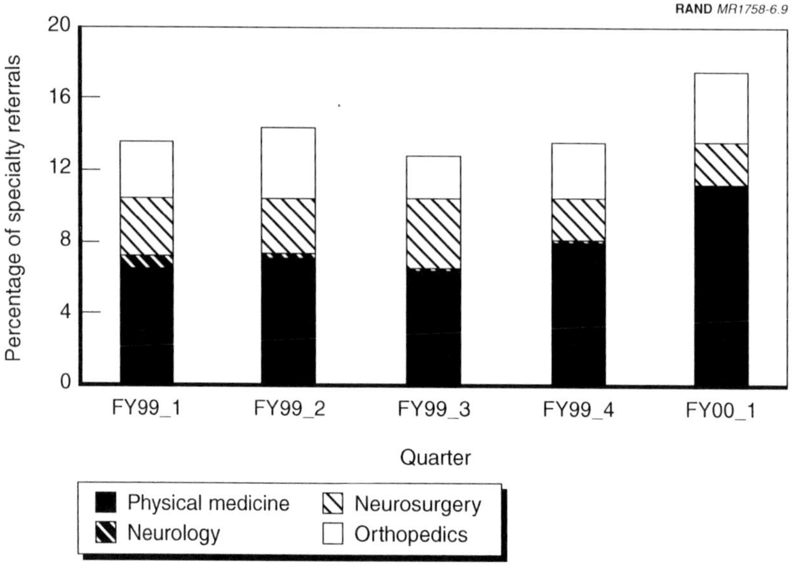

Figure 6.9—Trends in Distributions of Specialty Referrals for Acute Low Back Pain Patients by Type of Specialty, Demonstration Site D

there would be a reduction in use for the demonstration sites. However, we found no change in the prescribing of muscle relaxants during the demonstration. A total of 15,570 patients were prescribed muscle relaxants, and there were no observable trends in prescription rates over time for either demonstration or control sites or for any individual demonstration site (Table 6.6 and Figures 6.10 and 6.11). Statistical tests (see Appendix C) confirmed that trends for the demonstration and control sites were not significantly different. The absence of declines in use of muscle relaxants indicates that the demonstration sites did not address this provision of the guideline at all.

Table 6.6

Patients Prescribed Muscle Relaxants Within Six Weeks of Initial Low Back Pain Encounter, by MTF and Quarter

MTF Group	Number of Patients Prescribed	Percentage Prescribed 1st Qtr, 1999	2nd Qtr, 1999	3rd Qtr, 1999	4th Qtr, 1999	1st Qtr, 2000
Demonstration sites	7,507	46.8	43.8	46.6	47.4	45.9
Site A	3,558	56.7	42.6	54.1	49.4	47.6
Site B	991	36.3	40.0	36.3	44.6	45.4
Site C	1,568	34.7	39.4	36.1	41.5	41.5
Site D	1,390	50.9	55.7	47.3	53.0	49.6
Great Plains control sites	2,562	50.2	54.3	50.3	47.8	49.4
Site C1	644	45.1	46.2	43.3	42.5	46.1
Site C2	1,079	52.2	55.5	52.8	56.1	54.3
Site C3	839	51.3	59.8	54.3	42.8	46.6
Other control sites	5,501	55.7	55.1	53.2	56.0	58.1
Site C4	1,725	59.5	52.6	50.1	47.6	45.1
Site C5	3,776	53.7	56.3	55.0	60.2	64.5

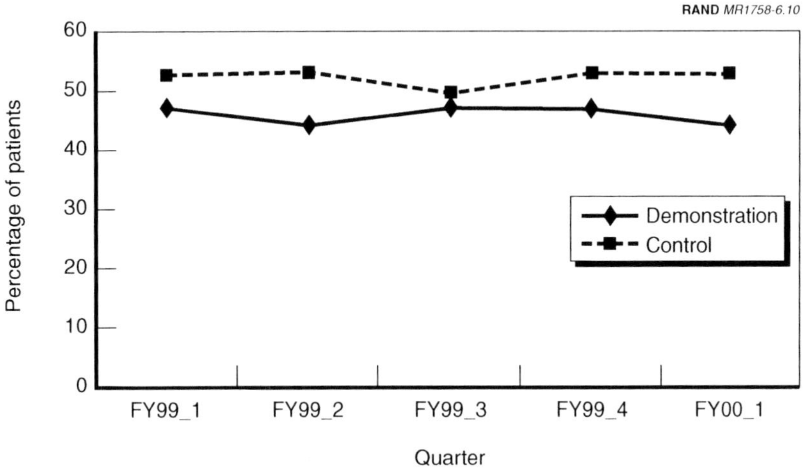

Figure 6.10—Percentage of Acute Low Back Pain Patients Prescribed Muscle Relaxants, at Demonstration and Control MTFs

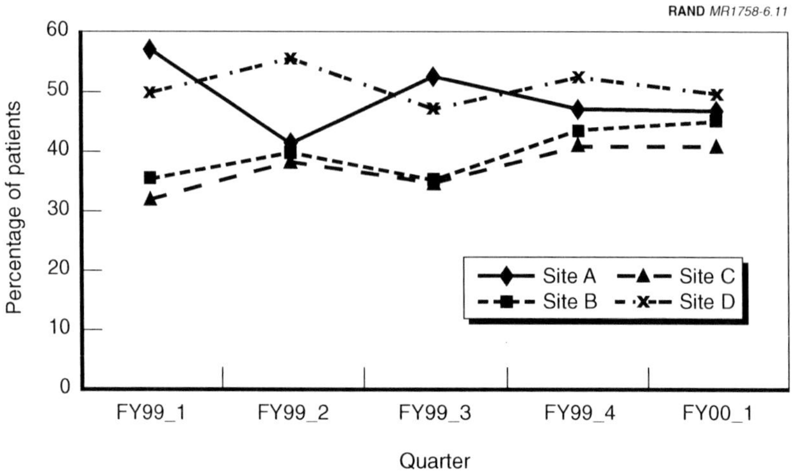

Figure 6.11—Percentage of Acute Low Back Pain Patients Prescribed Muscle Relaxants, by Demonstration MTF

Prescription of Narcotics

The low back pain guideline advises that NSAIDs should be the first line of pain control, with narcotics to be used only for cases of pain levels that NSAIDs cannot help. Given that an average of 33 percent of acute low back pain patients at the demonstration sites had been prescribed narcotics during the baseline period (see Chapter Three), we hypothesized there would be a decline in the percentage of patients prescribed narcotics during the conservative treatment period. A total of 10,113 low back pain patients were prescribed narcotics, representing almost one-third of the patients.

We found modest rates of reductions in narcotic prescription rates during the demonstration period for both the demonstration and control sites. This result indicates that providers' prescribing patterns were changing in the desired direction, as recommended by the guideline, but introduction of the guideline at the demonstration MTFs did not affect the trends at those sites (Table 6.7 and Figure 6.12). Statistical tests (see Appendix C) confirmed that trends for the

Table 6.7

Patients Prescribed Narcotics Within Six Weeks of Initial Low Back Pain Encounter, by MTF and Quarter

MTF Group	Number of Patients Prescribed	Percentage Prescribed				
		1st Qtr, 1999	2nd Qtr, 1999	3rd Qtr, 1999	4th Qtr, 1999	1st Qtr, 2000
Demonstration sites	5,016	33.3	31.4	31.8	29.7	27.6
Site A	2,252	34.9	29.9	33.7	31.3	28.4
Site B	834	35.5	35.4	30.3	35.3	32.6
Site C	992	25.6	25.7	26.9	22.8	22.2
Site D	938	38.5	38.7	33.4	31.2	30.4
Great Plains control sites	1,796	37.8	37.8	35.8	31.9	33.2
Site C1	545	39.4	40.4	38.7	36.3	34.2
Site C2	629	33.1	34.1	33.2	27.9	29.1
Site C3	622	42.2	40.6	36.2	32.7	37.1
Other control sites	3,401	37.9	37.3	31.5	34.2	30.9
Site C4	1,285	42.6	40.8	33.6	39.9	33.0
Site C5	2,116	35.3	35.6	30.4	31.4	29.8

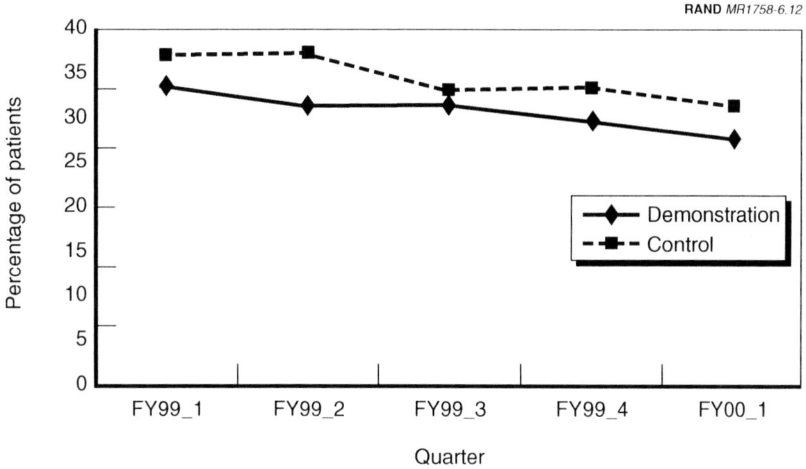

Figure 6.12—Percentage of Acute Low Back Pain Patients Prescribed Narcotics, for Demonstration and Control MTFs

demonstration and control sites were not significantly different. Of the four demonstration sites, Site C had the lowest narcotics prescription rates, and Site D had the largest reduction in narcotics prescriptions during the demonstration period (Figure 6.13).

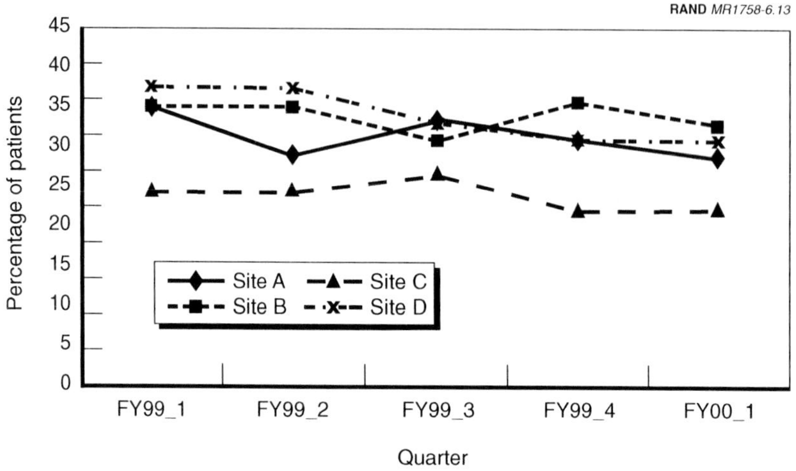

Figure 6.13—Percentage of Acute Low Back Pain Patients Prescribed Narcotics, by Demonstration MTF

Prescription of High-Cost NSAIDs

Although the low back pain guideline is silent regarding use of low-cost versus high-cost NSAIDs, the DoD PharmacoEconomic Center published materials documenting these cost differences and stating there were few differences in pain killing properties between the high- and low-cost NSAIDs.[1] These materials were included in the MEDCOM low back pain toolkit provided to the demonstration sites. With this information available to the sites, we hypothesized that use of high-cost NSAIDs at the demonstration sites would decline during the demonstration period.

---

[1]See Appendix A for the list of drugs classified as high-cost NSAIDs.

As shown in Table 6.8 and Figure 6.14 (and also the baseline data in Chapter Three), high-cost NSAID prescriptions were generally small percentages of the total NSAID prescriptions for patients at most demonstration and control sites. However, the percentages of high-cost NSAIDs increased substantially at one demonstration site (Site D) and moderately at one control site (Site C1) during the demonstration period (Table 6.8 and Figure 6.15). Also of note, the percentage of high-cost NSAIDs prescribed at one of the demonstration sites (Site C) steadily decreased in the period following introduction of the guideline, although this probably was coincidental because the site had not defined actions on this issue in its implementation action plan. We examined trends in use of high-cost NSAIDs for all the demonstration and control sites as well as for the two groups after removing episodes of care for patients at the two MTFs with increasing use of the high-cost NSAIDs (Figure 6.14). No significant change in the rate of prescription of high-cost NSAIDs is observed for the demonstration or control sites during the demonstration period, and statistical tests confirmed that trends for the demonstration and control sites were not significantly different (see Appendix C).

Table 6.8

High-Cost NSAIDs Prescribed Within Six Weeks of Initial Low Back Pain Encounter, by MTF and Quarter

MTF Group	High-Cost NSAID Prescriptions	Percentage of Total NSAID Prescriptions				
		1st Qtr, 1999	2nd Qtr, 1999	3rd Qtr, 1999	4th Qtr, 1999	1st Qtr, 2000
Demonstration sites	1,740	3.6	5.1	5.6	6.4	7.1
Site A	624	3.2	4.1	4.5	4.4	5.2
Site B	124	1.1	1.3	4.7	3.4	6.0
Site C	246	3.0	6.5	5.2	2.9	1.3
Site D	746	6.7	8.0	10.6	16.6	21.5
Great Plains control sites	456	2.3	3.0	4.8	5.1	6.2
Site C1	270	4.3	7.0	9.7	10.9	14.0
Site C2	62	0.6	1.6	2.7	0.6	2.0
Site C3	124	3.0	2.0	3.3	4.1	4.0
Other control sites	286	2.4	1.4	1.4	1.1	0.9
Site C4	146	3.0	2.8	1.7	2.0	1.0
Site C5	140	2.1	0.7	1.2	0.7	0.8

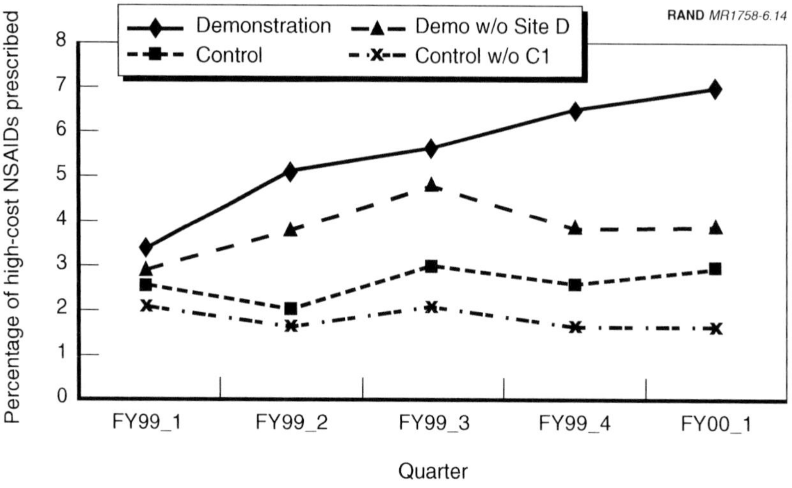

Figure 6.14—High-Cost NSAIDs Prescribed for Acute Low Back Pain Patients as a Percentage of All NSAIDs Prescribed, Demonstration and Control MTFs

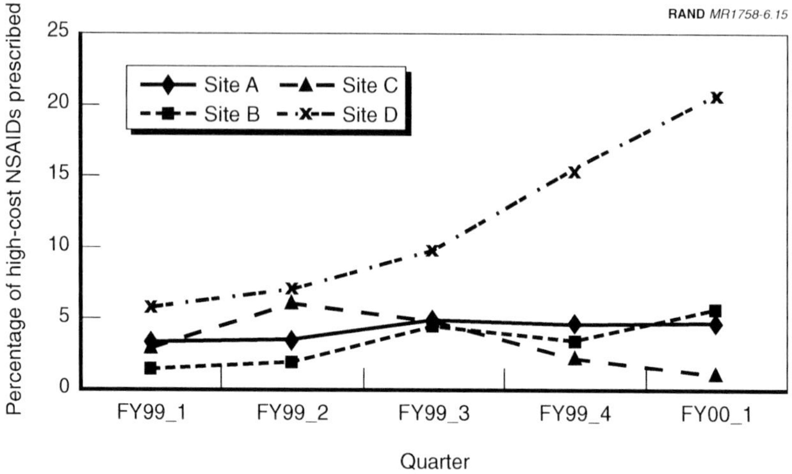

Figure 6.15—High-Cost NSAIDs Prescribed for Acute Low Back Pain Patients as a Percentage of All NSAIDs Prescribed, by Demonstration MTF

DISCUSSION

Our evaluation found that the perceptions of demonstration site participants about guideline effects on their practices were reasonably consistent with findings from our encounter data analysis, although some discrepancies did arise. For example, providers reported they increased physical therapy referrals, while some sites reported declines in referrals, and we found trends of declining referral rates in the encounter data. Others reported rates of follow-up visits that were consistent with those estimated from the encounter data. For pain medications, providers correctly reported no change in use of muscle relaxants, but their perceptions of use of NSAIDs and narcotics were not confirmed by the pharmacy data.

Most sites in this demonstration generated fairly limited objective data on their utilization trends, which precluded greater comparisons between such local data and the centralized encounter data (SADR, Standard Inpatient Data Record, and pharmacy data from the PharmacoEconomic Center). The local data were limited in part because low back pain metrics were not established until later in the demonstration. Other factors also contributed to limited monitoring by the sites, including competing demands for the implementation team members' time, mixed reactions by providers and clinic staff to using the guideline, and lack of mandates from MTF commands.

Effects of the demonstration on care for low back pain patients were limited during the first year the sites worked with the practice guideline, and effects that were found were for patterns of service delivery rather than for prescribing of pain medications. The only overall effect for the demonstration was a decline in physical therapy referrals during the demonstration period. The decline in numbers of follow-up primary care visits in the last quarter of the demonstration may be an early sign of a trend, but additional data for later months would be needed to verify such a trend was real. Despite not finding overall effects, effects were observed from the encounter data that were specific to individual sites and consistent with their implementation strategies. The strongest of these were the Site A strategy to use back classes to reduce use of physical therapy, which was observed in the data as declines in physical therapy referrals; and the Site D strategy to establish the physical medicine clinic as gatekeeper and reduce inappropriate specialty referrals, which were observed in the data as shifts of referrals to the physical medicine clinic from other specialties.

The implications of these evaluation findings for ongoing implementation of practice guidelines in AMEDD are considered in Chapter Seven.

Chapter Seven

LESSONS FROM THE LOW BACK PAIN DEMONSTRATION

This first demonstration to field test methods for implementation of clinical practice guidelines yielded rich information and insights even as it struggled to achieve lasting new practices. Despite disappointing results in terms of the effects on treatment of acute low back pain, the demonstration contributed to improvements in methods for subsequent guideline demonstrations, and ultimately, for implementation of the low back pain guideline in all Army health facilities as of the spring of 2000.

In this chapter, we synthesize the factors influencing the successes and limitations of the low back pain guideline demonstration. We begin by examining how well the demonstration performed on the six critical success factors presented in the beginning of this report and reintroduced throughout, and we assess how this performance contributed to the demonstration results. Then we identify a number of issues for the MTFs that emerged from the demonstration that are likely to affect other MTF guideline implementation efforts. Finally, we discuss implications for MEDCOM with respect to approaches and methods as it moves forward with implementation of a number of DoD/VA practice guidelines in the Army health system.

PERFORMANCE ON SIX CRITICAL SUCCESS FACTORS

Research on practice guideline implementation has documented that a commitment to the implementation process, including use of multiple interventions, is required to achieve desired changes to clinical practices. Below are the six critical success factors that are essential for making lasting changes in the MTFs' clinical and administrative processes. We discuss here the extent to which this demonstration realized these success factors, and we consider their effects on progress in implementing practice improvements.

1. **Command leadership commitment at the MTF, regional, and corporate levels.** This demonstration provides a meaningful example of how leadership commitment can affect the ability to achieve practice improvements. The regional leadership endorsed the demonstration strongly, but local commanders exhibited mixed levels of commitment, and changes in command eroded this support yet further over time. Given that this was the first demonstration in a new MEDCOM initiative, it is understandable that it might be met with mixed reactions due to concerns regarding the initiative's effects on MTF workloads and costs. Further, many providers, including physicians in leadership roles, have instinctive negative reactions to practice guidelines as "cookbook medicine," which indeed we heard in our evaluation. Unfortunately, passive or "wait and see" positions by command teams can become a self-fulfilling prophecy leading to failure because implementation teams are not given the motivation and support they need to change clinic procedures and mobilize providers and staff to accept the new practices. We believe these dynamics contributed to the limited results of the low back pain guideline demonstration.
2. **Monitoring of progress.** The demonstration did not perform well in the area of monitoring, in part because this was the first demonstration and it began very quickly as the DoD/VA practice guideline was being completed. The guideline expert panel did not select the key metrics for systemwide monitoring until well into the demonstration period. Further, MEDCOM did not have the resources early in this demonstration to establish a monitoring system at the corporate level. Without structured guidance from the corporate level, the sites varied widely in their approach to monitoring. One of the sites was quite aggressive in tracking utilization, but the other sites did not routinely monitor many measures. Some sites performed chart reviews to assess compliance with checking for red-flag conditions and documentation of

care, but these reviews were one-time events that were not established as regular monitoring mechanisms.

3. **Guidance and support to the MTFs by MEDCOM.** Within the limitations of available staff resources, MEDCOM made a solid commitment to provide the MTFs with policy guidance and technical support to enhance their ability to implement best practices for low back pain treatment. Such support can also encourage movement toward consistency in practices across the Army facilities. The nature of this support evolved during the demonstration, ultimately including preparation of a toolkit of support materials, hands-on technical support through site visits, and coordination of information exchange among the MTFs. Even though MEDCOM staff constraints led to some temporary delays in preparing the low back pain toolkit materials at the start of the demonstration, we believe MEDCOM's committed support has been a powerful foundation for the practice improvements achieved in the guideline demonstrations. MEDCOM learned from each field test and applied those lessons to subsequent demonstrations. Many of these lessons began with the low back pain demonstration.
4. **Guideline champions who are opinion leaders.** At the start of the low back pain demonstration, the participating MTFs identified well-respected physicians to serve as guideline champions, and all of these physicians showed a commitment to leading the implementation activities for their facilities. Some of the initial champions were lost to rotations and deployments, and they were replaced by other individuals. Each MTF's current status in implementing its action plan and its commitment to continued activities tended to influence its choice of a new champion, and it also affected the champion's sense of empowerment to achieve meaningful practice improvements. This demonstration revealed that champions are able to make only a time-limited commitment to such an initiative, after which they either "burn out" or must turn their attention to other priorities. Those who had leadership support worked harder and achieved more than those who did not. This finding highlights the importance of assimilating new practices as effectively and quickly as possible.
5. **Resource support for champions.** All of the MTF commanders authorized the champions to lead the implementation of the low

back pain guideline, but few of the champions received tangible resource support for their activities (other than attendance at the kickoff conference). Most of them had to perform the implementation work in addition to their regular workload. In most of the MTFs, a facilitator designated by the MTF commander provided some staff support to the champion, and for some, this role was an integral part of the facilitator's regular job. Provision of additional resources to support implementation activities would have helped the champion and team to achieve lasting improvements in practices.

6. **Institutionalization of new practices.** Three of the participating MTFs made early progress in achieving practices consistent with the low back pain guideline. The fourth MTF had defined few actions to change practices, reflecting its view that low back pain care was a low-priority quality issue. Two of the sites that pursued implementation activities lost momentum over time, one because of heavy workload demands related to deployments and the other because of changing priorities associated with changes in command. Only one site achieved practice changes that are likely to remain in place, including the establishment of the physical medicine clinic as gatekeeper and new procedures to handle specialty referrals. These changes have a good chance of surviving because they addressed an issue that was important to providers and MTF leadership. It is a major challenge to achieve new practices that are resistant to the destabilizing effects of staff turnover or shifts in policies at the command level. This issue became a focus of the asthma and diabetes demonstrations, with the goal of identifying successful techniques.

Although the MTFs in all the demonstrations were generally successful in identifying effective champion leaders, there was a consistent absence of dedicated time to help these champions perform their additional roles. In addition, MTF command commitment was only moderate in general, and it varied across MTFs and regions from somewhat passive support to active opposition. Several changes in commanders also occurred that had negative effects on command support. These limitations have contributed to weakening the teams' ability to change the way low back pain was managed in their facilities and, thus, contributed to the effects of their activities on the clinical practice indicators and other desired outcomes.

As intended in the original project design, the experiences of this demonstration helped us identify a number of improvements for the asthma and diabetes demonstrations, with resulting improvements in performance on many of the six success factors. The most noticeable improvements were gained in the monitoring of implementation progress by the MTFs and in the amount and timeliness of MEDCOM support to the MTFs. MEDCOM support was strengthened as additional staff were hired to work with the MTFs on multiple guideline implementation activities.

SOME PERSPECTIVES FOR THE TREATMENT FACILITIES

As we observed the experiences of the participating MTFs during the demonstration, we identified several challenges that MTFs are likely to face regularly in implementation efforts. By recognizing and preparing to manage these challenges, MTFs can better achieve their goals in implementing practice guidelines or other quality improvement activities:

- Momentum (or lack of it) will strongly influence progress in achieving new practices. Therefore, teams should strive to achieve early successes that capitalize on the momentum generated by the start-up activities when the team is defining problems and preparing its action plan.
- Although command leadership commitment is necessary for changing clinical practices, it is not a sufficient ingredient. Achievement of goals will also require follow-through by the implementation team in carrying out actions and monitoring progress.
- The best chance of establishing lasting new clinic procedures requires the sincere involvement of all clinic staff. It is worth taking the time required to educate all potential participants about the goals and contents of a guideline and to build their understanding and acceptance of the best practices being introduced.
- Even the most well designed and executed action plan will not be able to change the practices of all patients and providers. Ongoing monitoring and maintenance interventions will be needed to

continue progress toward full compliance with practice standards by all those involved in the care delivery process.

- Among the first actions that should be taken in implementing new practices are to define the metrics for monitoring and to work with the appropriate offices to get the necessary data. Ideally, the implementation team should establish the capability to provide monitoring feedback to its MTF clinics within a month or two after beginning implementation of new clinical practices.
- Rotations of personnel are an ongoing part of military life, and they should not be an excuse for lack of progress on implementing improved practices. As each MTF defines its action plan and schedule, it should anticipate and plan for military rotations, including effects on the clinic staff and on the members of the implementation team itself. Any surprise personnel movements that affect staffing can be accommodated by action plan updates and revisions.

THE CORPORATE PERSPECTIVE

Guided by the experiences of the low back pain demonstration, as well as by the asthma and diabetes guideline demonstrations, a corporate implementation strategy emerged that was found to be an effective and efficient approach for practice guideline implementation in AMEDD. The field experience bore out the value of a systems approach, in this case including both corporate and local roles as well as application of multiple implementation actions within each MTF. Continuous quality improvement techniques served well in planning and carrying out the implementation steps. These steps are (1) preparation of a realistic action plan by each MTF that defines a focused strategy and sets of actions to introduce the guideline and to change clinic procedures (where needed), (2) performance of the defined actions by designated staff, (3) ongoing monitoring of progress in making intended practice changes through the actions undertaken, and (4) adjustment of action strategies in response to monitoring findings. This process is based on the recognition that quality improvement involves a series of manageable, incremental steps, each of which builds on previous steps over time to achieve continual improvements in health care processes and outcomes.

We list here some items that arose from the low back pain demonstration, which are within the authority and responsibility of MEDCOM. Careful attention to the following should help build an effective program to support the MTFs in their implementation activities:

- Commit corporate leadership to implementation of evidence-based best practices, which is essential to establishing a viable program across the AMEDD system. This support sets the tone for activities at all levels of the organization.
- Maintain the proactive role of MEDCOM in managing a coordinated guideline implementation program across the system, including the responsiveness MEDCOM has shown to MTFs as they have pursued local implementation activities. MEDCOM has eased the workload for MTFs by providing tools and technical guidance, thus enhancing the potential to achieve practice improvements.
- When introducing a new practice guideline for MTF implementation, provide clear guidance and instructions so the MTFs know what is expected of them and where they have the flexibility to act locally. Set objectives and define what is mandated and what is left to MTF discretion. Maintain a balance between flexibility for local MTF approaches and provision of sufficient policy direction to ensure that AMEDD is moving toward greater consistency in practices.
- Move forward strongly on establishment of a system-level monitoring process to track MTF progress in improving clinical practices. This function should develop the data and analytic capability to perform the measurement and report results to the MTFs, and it also should be equipped to provide training and support to MTFs for their local monitoring processes.
- Provide resources to support implementation activities at levels commensurate with the expected workload and results, including resources for both MEDCOM and the MTFs.
- Reevaluate the MEDCOM policy on the use of standard forms in the management of care for conditions addressed by the practice guidelines. Although the low back pain documentation form was shown to improve provider efficiency, it became a point of con-

tention that often distracted from the real task at hand—the improvement of low back pain care. The number of new forms will multiply as more guidelines are introduced, which could be a deterrent for the program if not presented appropriately.

- Develop contractual mechanisms to ensure that contract providers participate in implementing improved practices. Contract providers resisted participation for the low back pain guideline, and similar resistance was observed in other demonstrations. These attitudes are due in part to financial incentives created by their contracts, where they are paid based on the number of visits they complete, and time spent on any other activities is unpaid time.
- Provide proactive MEDCOM leadership for ensuring full information exchange among MTFs. Individual MTFs are not likely to take the lead in communicating information or ideas with others because each of them has a full set of work commitments that tend to discourage it from looking beyond the MTF boundaries.
- Provide guidance and training to the MTFs on how to perform effective patient education as part of the treatment of conditions covered by practice guidelines, including techniques for encouraging patients to assume greater responsibility for self-care.
- Pay attention to the details of the diversity of issues the MTFs raise as they work with a guideline. Examples of issues that occurred in the low back pain demonstration (as well as later in the asthma and diabetes guideline demonstrations) include how to handle patients presenting with multiple concerns or diagnoses, placement of documentation forms in the medical chart, procedures for use of diagnostic codes for visits, and the reading level for patient education materials.
- Managing care according to the DoD/VA practice guidelines represents a proactive primary care management approach for patients with specific health conditions. Thus, consider replacing traditional utilization review functions with this more proactive approach to achieve appropriate and consistent practices.

Resource limitations inevitably define the scope of implementation any given MTF can undertake. Priorities for action should be consistent with available resources, and in turn, the needed resources should be provided to support the agreed-upon actions. Both the actions defined and the allocation of resources should be *time limited,* so that the desired new practices can be successfully integrated into a clinic's routine and then these resources can be reallocated to other priorities.

Appendix A

EVALUATION METHODOLOGY

PROCESS EVALUATION

To capture the full dynamics of a process as complex as practice guideline implementation, it is important to take into account the roles and interactions of the many aspects of the system in which the guidelines are being implemented. Figure A.1 is a diagram of relationships among the different levels of a health care organization during guideline implementation, the stakeholders involved, and the dynamics of the implementation process.

A variety of stakeholders need to be considered to ensure that individuals involved in implementing new practices anticipate possible effects on the stakeholders and responses that might be expected from them. These groups include treatment program leadership, middle management, the clinical and administrative staff working with program residents, and the clients themselves. The implementation team consists of important stakeholders who not only are serving as team members but also have other job responsibilities.

Information was collected about the actions involved in practice guideline implementation for participating MTFs, the dynamics of the change process, and responses of participants to their experiences with the process. Similarities and differences in the attitudes, motivations, and preferences of the stakeholders were considered as the process evaluation information was collected and results were synthesized. To capture changes in structures, processes, and issues as guideline implementation moved forward, site visits were conducted to collect information at baseline and at two follow-up times, as shown in Table A.1.

A participant-observer approach was used throughout the implementation process and evaluation. In addition to the site visits, we used routine progress reports and maintained an ongoing communication process to provide a structure through which implementing MTFs could get assistance from each other, MEDCOM, or RAND.

Both qualitative and quantitative data collection methods were used in the process evaluation to collect information on a set of questions that cover the dimensions shown in Table A.1. Shown in Table A.2 are the specific topic areas covered and relevant data collection methods.

RAND *MR1758-A.1*

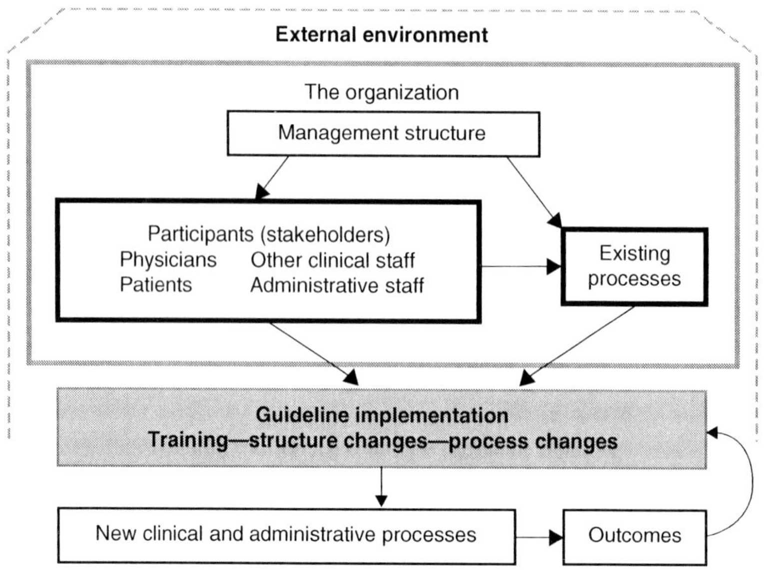

Figure A.1—A System View of Guideline Implementation

Table A.1

Dimensions Addressed by the Process Evaluation

	Baseline	Month 3	Month 9
Structure and organization	X	X	X
Culture and climate	X		X
Current practices	X	X	X
Environmental context	X	X	X
Stakeholders' attitudes	X	X	X
Implementation plan		X	X
Changes in clinic processes		X	X
AMEDD support systems		X	X
Staff involvement		X	X
Patient roles and reactions		X	X
Monitoring progress		X	X
Effects on stakeholders		X	X

Interviews and focus groups with the implementation team, providers and clinic staff, quality management staff, and other participants yielded information on the dynamics of the implementation process. Focus groups were conducted with three groups: the implementation team, providers, and other clinic staff. Participants in each stakeholder group were asked questions regarding their attitudes toward guideline implementation, how they worked with the practice guideline, how they were affected by the implementation process, and issues or concerns they identified. Semi-structured interview methods were used for all interviews, group discussions, and focus groups, working from lists of questions to cover during each session.

A brief survey regarding stakeholders' attitudes toward practice guidelines and quality improvement processes was administered at baseline and the final site visit. The survey at the final site visit also included questions about education received on the guideline, actions taken to implement the new practices, and how those actions affected providers and clinic staff.

Documents and materials were also important sources of information for the process evaluation. These included written information about the MTF structure and management, MTF policies and procedures, MTF data collection and monitoring, and materials developed by the MTF implementation teams as they prepared and carried out

Table A.2

Dimensions Addressed by the Process Evaluation and Data Collection Methods

	Document Materials	Monitor Reports	Individual Interviews[a]	Focus Groups	Culture Survey
Environmental context					
How supportive was culture and climate					X
How did culture and climate change					X
Other factors affecting implementation			X	X	
The implementation plan					
What key guideline elements are priorities	X	X	X	X	
What information is used to identify priorities			X	X	
How is guideline team organized	X		X	X	
How does guideline team operate			X	X	
How was guideline introduced to staff	X	X	X	X	
Planned changes to processes					
What process changes did MTFs identify	X	X	X	X	
Which changes did MTFs implement		X	X	X	
What factors supported or slowed changes		X	X	X	
How were implementation plans changed	X	X	X	X	
AMEDD systems for implementation					
Help from MEDCOM on implementation		X	X	X	
How useful was implementation toolkit		X	X	X	
How useful were KMN and communications		X	X	X	
Help from MEDCOM on monitoring methods		X	X	X	

Table A.2—continued

	Document Materials	Monitor Reports	Individual Interviews[a]	Focus Groups	Culture Survey
Clinical and administrative staff effects					
Attitudes of MDs and other staff at the start			X	X	X
MD and other staff roles in implementation			X	X	
MDs motivated to adopt new practices			X	X	
Effects of changes on MDs and responses					
Effects on other staff workload and demands					
Roles and reactions of patients					
Patients' responses to changes in care			X	X	
How team managed patient reactions			X	X	
Helpfulness of patient education materials			X	X	
Effects on physician-patient relationship			X	X	
Measuring implementation progress					
Indicators the MTF selected for monitoring	X	X			
MTF data system for monitoring	X	X	X	X	
Lessons from monitoring and actions taken		X	X	X	
Usefulness of monitoring to clinical staff			X	X	

[a]Individual interviews included one-on-one interviews and written questionnaires completed by key participants.

their action plans to changes practices. The materials provided the primary documentation on the actions planned by the team, changes made to clinic processes, resulting events, and actions taken to monitor their progress.

EVALUATION OF EFFECTS (OUTCOMES)

Indicators selected for the evaluation of guideline effects were those that could be measured using available administrative data on health care encounters, use of prescription medications, and the demographic and clinical characteristics of the clients. These measures were estimated based on episodes of treatment for acute low back pain that began with an initial clinic visit for low back pain and continued through a subsequent six-week time period. According to the DoD/VA low back pain guideline, this six-week period represents acute low back pain, and pain continuing after that period is considered to be chronic low back pain. The guideline recommends use of conservative treatment for acute low back pain.

Identifying Initial Outpatient Visits for Low Back Pain

1. For a specified quarter year (three-month period), we extracted all SADR encounter records that (a) were coded as active duty Army personnel, (b) had a code of 722 (intervertebral disc disorders) or 724 (other and unspecified disorders of back) in any diagnostic code field, and (c) were treated at one of the MTFs included in the analysis.
2. We deleted from the data set any record that was coded as no-show, canceled by facility, canceled by patient, left without being seen, or telephone consult (APPTMNT Status = 6).
3. When two or more encounter records were found for an individual during the quarter, we retained only the record with the earliest "start date" of service.
4. We deleted any encounter record containing one of the following codes:
    - Clinic code of BCC (obstetrics), BEE (orthotics), BFD (psychiatry), or BLA (physical therapy).
    - Provider class code of CN (clinical nursing), PT (physical therapy), or OUT (outside provider).
    - Specialty code of 706 (physical therapist).

5. For records with missing specialty and provider class codes, we retained those with clinic codes of BAA, BIA, BGA, BHA, and BJA (all primary care clinics).

6. For each candidate "initial visit" in the resulting data set, we searched for any SADR encounter records for that patient that occurred within 90 days before the date of service on the candidate visit record and that had diagnostic codes of 722 or 724. Any candidate "initial visit" record for a patient with such an earlier encounter was deleted from the study.

Building Analysis Files with Data on Low Back Pain Episodes and Patients

Data on subsequent clinical encounters and pharmaceuticals for patients' low back pain episodes were extracted from the SADR, USPD, and SIDPERS source files. Data from these three sources can be merged using the patient Social Security number. The focus could be on conservative treatment during the acute care phase (first six weeks after initial low back pain visit) or the chronic care phase (up to six months after the initial visit). Although we extracted data for encounters up to six months after the initial visit, we focused on the acute care phase for this evaluation. The following records were extracted for all initial patient visits:

- All SADR encounter records for a six-month time period following the initial visit, regardless of the health care facility where the patient obtained care.[1]
- All USPD records of pharmaceuticals filled in MTF pharmacies for a six-month time period following the initial visit, regardless of the health care facility where the patient obtained care.
- Variables from the Army SIDPERS file to identify patient characteristics of age, gender, and military rank.

---

[1]For this analysis, the treatment files were extracted only from the MTFs involved in the demonstration project, rather than extracting all of the patients' encounters at any MTFs. We believe the missing data do not affect our results because all but a very small percentage of active duty personnel would obtain acute low back pain care at the MTFs where they are currently posted (this is less likely to be the case for chronic low back pain care).

Definition of Key Variables

The measures of effects of the low back pain guideline demonstration included three types of service utilization (clinic visits) and three measures for utilization of pain medications. In addition, military rank, age, and gender were used to control for patient characteristics in modeling effects of the demonstration. Table A.3 shows the coding that was used to define each variable.

Table A.3

Coding Variables

Variable	Codes Used for the Definition
Physical therapy or chiropractic visit	A visit in a clinic with a three-digit MEPRS[a] code of BLA (physical therapy clinic) or BEZ (orthopedic care not elsewhere), a provider specialty code of 706 (PT), or a provider class code of PT
Primary care visit	A visit in a clinic with a three-digit MEPRS code of BGA (family practice clinic), BHA (primary care clinic), BJA (flight medicine clinic), or BAA (internal medicine clinic)
Neurology visit	A visit in a clinic with a three-digit MEPRS code of BAK or with a provider specialty code of 060 (neurologist)
Neurosurgery visit	A visit in a clinic with a three-digit MEPRS code of BBC or with a provider specialty code of 106 (neurosurgeon)
Physical medicine and rehabilitation	A visit in a clinic with a three-digit MEPRS code of BAR (physical medicine clinic) or BBL (pain management clinic) or with a provider specialty code of 090 (physical medicine physician) or 950 (physical medicine and rehabilitation)
Orthopedics visit	A visit in a clinic with a three-digit MEPRS code of BEA or with a provider specialty code of 140 (orthopedic surgeon) or 947 (orthopedics)
Specialty care visit	A visit in a clinic with any of the three-digit MEPRS codes or with provider specialty codes listed for the neurology, neurosurgery, physical medicine and rehabilitation, or orthopedics visits
Muscle relaxant	Generic drug names of Cyclobenzaprine HCL, Diazepam, Methocarbamol, Chlorzoxazone, Carisoprodol, Metaxalone, or one of the orphenadrines
Low-cost NSAID	Generic drug names of Salsalate, Ibuprofen, Indomethacin, Naproxen, Naproxen Sodium, Piroxicam, Sulindac, or one of the cholines

Table A.3—continued

Variable	Codes Used for the Definition
High-cost NSAID	Generic drug names of Diflusinal, Etodolac, Ketoprophen, Fluribiprofen Sodium, Meclofenamate Sodium, Mefenamic Acid, Tolmetin Sodium, Celecoxib, Rofecoxib, Ketorolac Tromethamine, Nabumetone, Oxaprizin, or one of the diclofenacs
Any NSAID	Defined as either a low-cost or high-cost NSAID
Narcotic	Generic drug names of Codeine Phosphate, Codeine Sulfate, Codeine with Acetaminophen, Morphine Sulfate, one of the hydrocodones, one of the oxycodones, one of the pentazocines, or one of the propoxyphenes
Rank of active duty personnel	Officer (ranks of 20 to 29), warrant (ranks of 10 to 15), or enlisted (ranks of 1 to 9), based on coding in the SIDPERS data. An alternative variable was also defined that collapsed the officer and warrant officer rank into one officer category
Patient age	Categories of age less than 30 years, 30 to 39 years, or 40 years or older

[a]Medical Expense and Performance Report System for Fixed Military Medical and Dental Treatment Facilities.

To be considered part of an episode of low back pain care, a follow-up outpatient MTF visit had to occur within six weeks after the initial visit and include a diagnosis code relevant to low back pain. For the physical therapy or manipulation visits and the follow-up primary care visits, all encounters with the low back pain codes of 722 or 724 were defined as relevant visits. For specialty care visits, we expanded the list of diagnosis codes to include other relevant conditions or complications associated with low back pain that might require specialty care.[2] Medications were considered to be part of an episode of low back pain care if they were included in the definitions of muscle relaxants, narcotics, or NSAIDs and the prescription fill date occurred within six weeks after the initial visit.

---

[2]The additional specialty visit diagnosis codes were 307.89, 344.6, 355.0, 716.98, 720.0–721.9, 723.0–723.9, 729.0, 729.1, 729.2, 732.0, 732.8, 733.00–733.13, 737.0–737.9, 846.0–846.9, 847.1–847.4, 847.9, and V65.2.

Appendix B

REPORTS FROM THE FINAL ROUND OF SITE VISITS

This appendix contains the site visit reports that present findings from RAND's second round of evaluation visits to the four Army MTFs participating in the demonstration to implement the DoD/VA practice guideline, *Primary Care Management of Low Back Pain.* These site visits were conducted during March and April 2000. During each site visit, the RAND team collected information from the MTF participants about their implementation activities using individual interviews, group discussions, and focus group methods. A structured agenda was established for each site visit in collaboration with the guideline facilitator and champion. Through the site visits, we learned the successes and challenges the sites experienced during their implementation processes, and we obtained feedback from participants regarding actions to improve the systemwide implementation of the practice guideline.

Since this demonstration was the first of three that were conducted by AMEDD and RAND in their partnership to field test methods for effective implementation of new evidence-based practices, the asthma and the diabetes demonstrations gained from the lessons learned from the low back pain guideline demonstration. This first demonstration allowed the incremental building of a more effective program to achieve reduction in clinical practice variation by introducing consistent, evidence-based practices. The site visits were as follows:

- *Site A—Site Visit on February 9–10, 2000.* Conducted by Georges Vernez and RAND Army Health Fellow COL George Dydek. LTC

Kathryn Dolter, from MEDCOM, and Charles Miller, MD, a MEDCOM consultant, accompanied them.

- *Site B—Site Visit on March 15–16, 2000.* Conducted by Georges Vernez and RAND Army Health Fellow MAJ Andre Marinkovich. Charles Miller, MD, a MEDCOM consultant, accompanied them.
- *Site C—Visit on February 7–8, 2000.* Conducted by Georges Vernez and RAND Army Health Fellow COL George Dydek. LTC Kathryn Dolter, from MEDCOM, and Charles Miller, MD, a MEDCOM consultant, accompanied them.
- *Site D—Site Visit on March 13–14, 2000.* Conducted by Georges Vernez and RAND Army Health Fellow MAJ Andre Marinkovich. Charles Miller, MD, a MEDCOM consultant, accompanied them.

SITE A

Overview of the Site Visit

Hampered by deployments and other high-priority demands on staff time, Site A did not undertake any new implementation activities since the three-month site visit in June 1999. Emphasis continued to be placed on educating patients on self-care for their low back pain. The participating clinics put in place new patient education referral processes, which have increased access in terms of location and frequency, with varying degrees of success. The QM/UM office is keeping track of the frequency of visits by low back pain patients and has reviewed charts to assess compliance with the practice guideline. The findings suggest there was a low rate of documentation of checking for red-flag conditions. Orthopedic providers also report no reduction in inappropriate (too early) referrals to this specialty.

The Organizational Context

In excess of 600 low back pain patients are seen monthly at the MTF's six outpatient clinics and three TMCs. The large number of clinics in dispersed locations has made it difficult for the implementation team to communicate effectively. Frequent deployments and the priority given to them by health care personnel have also affected continuity of effort for implementing the low back pain guideline. At any given time during the past year, up to 60 percent of providers were absent because of deployments and other assignments.

Another factor that hampered the ability to establish and maintain new practices was rotations of medics between clinics and the field units, which occurs every 80 to 90 days at Site A. Thus, an emphasis needs to be placed on ongoing education on the guideline and on continuity of effort. The MTF also has a relatively high share of contractors among its providers. Actions to ensure ongoing training of medics and contract providers have not been fully established yet.

The low back pain champion was particularly affected by competing demands for his time. His department lost several staff, with the result that he had to give priority to patient care. He estimated that 25–30 percent of his time should have been dedicated to implementation of the low back pain guideline, which he was unable to do. He believes that a guideline champion must have "protected time" from other duties to work on implementation.

Attitudes Toward the Low Back Pain Guideline

The attitudes of providers and ancillary staff toward the low back pain guideline continued to be generally positive. According to participants in the site visit, the guideline "provides specific guidance, for the first time, for when to refer a patient for more definitive diagnostic procedures," and it also provides "an effective way to quickly evaluate patients." The low back pain guideline is also valued as a reminder of good practices. The red-flag conditions were singled out as being extremely useful for appropriately triaging patients, particularly in the ER. Ancillary staff found the guideline "beneficial to explain the problem and treatment plan to patients." As in our earlier visit, our respondents identified no specific problems with the logic and content of the guideline. There was consensus, however, that a greater effort should be made on prevention of low back pain in the field, most particularly in basic training and in physical training.

There are notable exceptions to this positive feedback, however. Some physicians and PAs, mostly from TMCs, consider the guideline "cookbook medicine" and will not use it.

Implementation Activities

Implementation Strategy. The overall strategy that Site A defined for implementing the low back pain guideline had not changed since it was first developed at the kickoff conference. Site A's focus was on improving care for active duty personnel with acute low back pain, emphasizing patient education and self-care. The long-term goal was to prevent recurrence of low back pain episodes and reduce the need for referrals to specialists. Consistent with this approach, the main focus of changes in practices was to increase access and referrals of patients to back classes. Actions related to other components of the guideline tended to be left to the discretion of providers in the various clinics and TMCs.

Implementation Team. With one exception, the implementation team for the low back pain guideline remained the same as the one that attended the kickoff meeting. The exception was a new facilitator—an Army staff person who replaced the civilian who had served as facilitator since the start of the demonstration. The implementation team has 19 members, with one or two representatives from each clinic or TMC, one representative each from the operations and deployment medicine branch and PT, three representatives from QM/QI, and the champion. About one-half of this implementation team is expected to rotate to other assignments in the summer of 2000. To the extent that the team intended to continue operating past that time, the loss of personnel could compromise its viability.

The implementation team proved difficult to manage because of the large number of members and their decentralized locations. The team had not met in the past six months. Communications between members were limited to exchanges through email or CHCS. The result was a systemic breakdown in communications over time. For example, many team members were unaware of the changes made to the MEDCOM documentation form 695-R, methods for ordering additional brochures on patient self-care, the availability of information about the guideline on the MEDCOM QM web page, and the availability of the standard profile form developed at another demonstration site. In addition, the champion and other team members were not aware of CME opportunities for provider education on the low back pain guideline. These examples raise questions regarding communication within the Site A implementation team, as well as between MEDCOM and the demonstration sites.

Provider and Ancillary Staff Education. An initial effort was made in the spring of 1999 to train existing providers on the low back pain guideline, after which no further education was provided for newly arrived providers or for retraining of existing providers. In addition, ancillary staff were not provided any training or orientation on the guideline, even though the site had identified a need for such training during our first evaluation site visit. Thus, subsequent to the initial provider training on practices recommended by the guideline, whatever the new providers and ancillary staff learned about the guideline was obtained strictly through on-the-job training.

Respondents to our survey at the site visit were unanimous in recognizing that a capacity for ongoing provider *and* ancillary staff education was the key to successful implementation of any guideline.

The low back pain champion reported that he simply did not have the needed time to undertake the task, despite understanding how important it was to provide this education. The implementation team saw introduction of guidelines at graduate medical education schools as a key to successful implementation of guidelines in the long term.

Changes in Administrative Processes. Clinics and TMCs at Site A had to make "minor adjustments" to their routine procedures to include use of documentation form 695-R in processing patients during clinic visits. Two clinics and one TMC reported that, at the front desk, they hand the form 695-R to patients coming in for low back pain and ask them to fill it out prior to going to the screening room. In another clinic, however, medics had patients fill out form 695-R in the screening room. Ancillary staff reported that use of the form did not hinder the processing of patients and did not add time to their screening. However, they reported that providers were mixed in their actual use of form 695-R. In an audit of 98 low back pain patient charts, performed between May and December 1999, they found that an overall 58 percent of charts contained documentation form 695-R, but that percentages of charts with forms varied across clinics from a low of 7 percent to a high of 92 percent. Generally, TMCs were more likely to have the form included in charts than were MTF clinics.

Providers expressed dissatisfaction with the form during our first site visit, and they made several suggestions for improvements, including the need for more open space to write notes on the form. Although MEDCOM revised the form according to the suggestions from the four demonstration sites, Site A providers were unaware of the revised form, and, hence, many providers continued to be reluctant to use the form. Some staff reported that the form was perceived as a "test" form and suggested that it would not be widely used until it became mandatory.

At the time of our final visit, referrals of patients to back classes were treated as a consult. Those who are scheduled for a class have an SF-600 printed out and included in their medical records. Those who sign up for a class but fail to attend have their preprinted SF-600 stamped "NO SHOW." However, there was no process in place to follow up on referrals who elect not to sign up for the class or who sign up but do not attend. Some clinic staff were able to personally appeal to unit commanders to enforce participation in back classes. The chart audit referred to above showed that 54 percent of the low back pain patients sampled had been referred to a back class. Referral rates varied across clinics and TMCs from a low of 29 percent to a high of 76 percent. Also, before the guideline was introduced, and before emphasis was given to patient education, 25–30 percent of the referrals to PT had not attended a back class. As of February 2000, all patients must be referred to a back class before going to PT.

The Site A team raised two other procedural issues. The first concerned rules regarding where the documentation form 695-R should be placed in the patient's chart. Ancillary staff suggested the forms be placed in chronological order but were seeking some guidance from MEDCOM on this issue. Placing the documentation form into the charts of active duty personnel had not been perceived as an issue at our first visit, because active duty personnel are required to hand in their medical charts at the facility they are assigned to upon arrival. However, 59 percent of charts were found to be missing in the audit sample of low back pain patients, suggesting that this problem affects this site as much as any other Army MTF.

The second issue concerned the continuing use of two different ICD-9 diagnostic codes for low back pain despite MEDCOM's determination that one single code (724.2) was to be used for all low back pain visits. In fact, the site printed the two codes it decided to use on documentation form 695-R: 724.2 for acute or chronic low back pain and 724.3 for acute or chronic sciatica. This is another illustration of some gaps in communications between MEDCOM and this demonstration site and among members of the implementation team at the site.

Patient Education. The back classes for patients are offered at most of the clinics and TMCs. Their scheduling varies from weekly to once a month, depending on the volume of referrals, availability of personnel, and availability of space at the respective facilities. All respondents during our site visit expressed satisfaction with access to and the content of these classes.

At the clinic we visited, back classes were scheduled regularly every second and fourth Wednesday of the month. A very enthusiastic instructor leads these classes, using the material developed by the PT staff. She discusses the common causes of back problems and injuries including poor posture, poor body mechanics, lack of exercise, being overweight, diet, and smoking. She shows a video (either the MEDCOM video or one developed locally) and reviews the stretching and strengthening exercises shown on the handouts, which she leaves with the patients. Her class can accommodate 25 patients at a time. The no-show rate is about 25 percent.

One key factor that affects back class attendance is the willingness of unit commanders to allow soldiers to attend the classes. MTF staff have worked individually with commanders to resolve this issue, but no systematic approach has been taken. Some site visit participants perceived that attendance in back classes had decreased over time. However, this perception may be due to the increased availability of classes at other clinics and times that may be more convenient to patients rather than to a real decline in the number of patients attending classes. No organized effort had yet been undertaken to monitor class attendance and report rates back to the clinics.

At our first visit to Site A, the staff described various ideas they were considering to increase referrals and attendance to back classes. These included coordinating classes among clinics and sending patients to the first available class; renaming back class "physical therapy class" to indicate to the patient that it is a component of treatment; and working with primary care providers to increase "marketing" of back classes. There were apparently no actions taken to pursue these ideas.

Table B.1 presents the feedback on the toolkits provided to Site A MTFs.

Metrics and Monitoring

Site A monitored two different sets of metrics:

- number of low back pain patients and visits and number of visits per patient, total and per clinic, using ADS data
- presence of documentation form 695-R, documentation of referral to back class, and documentation that the red flags had been checked, using review of a sample of low back pain patients' charts.

Table B.1

Site A Assessment of Toolkit Items

Tool	Feedback from the Site
Video for CME	No additional use made of the CME video since our last visit. At that time, providers rated it "excellent."
MEDCOM documentation form 695-R	Positive comments: efficient tool to process patients, good for monitoring severity of patient problem, red-flag boxes useful for triaging patients, excellent to help discuss patients' low back pain problem and monitor patients' progress, potential to track soldiers' occupation and units to identify low back pain injury risks. Some prefer to use the form for the initial visit exclusively and not at all visits. Not helpful for visits where patients have multiple problems.
Patient education video	Rated "excellent" by all who saw it.
Patient education brochure	Rated "excellent" by all who saw it.
Key elements cards	No comments offered.
Standardized profile	Staff had not known of this addition to the toolkit. No comments offered.
Additional toolkit items	Staff suggested that posters directed at patients emphasizing prevention of low back pain injuries should be developed and placed in the work place as well as the clinics.

During the period from May 1, 1999, to December 17, 1999, the MTF and TMCs provided 6,924 visits for low back pain. Nearly one-half of these visits (47 percent) were one-time-only visits. In addition, there were about 900 visits to the ER for low back pain. Overall, there were 1.5 clinic visits per low back pain patient during this period. For patients who had more than one visit, the number of visits was 2.7 visits per patient. The average number of visits varied across the clinics and TMCs, ranging from 1.32 to 1.72 visits per patient. In general, TMCs had higher numbers of visits per patient than the MTF clinics.

This monitoring also identified a small number of patients (six) with greater than 10 visits. The implementation team plans to follow up on these patients to identify the reasons for such high utilization.

For the chart review, the implementation team attempted to pull the medical records for a sample of 391 low back pain patients with a visit between May 1, 1999, and November 2, 1999. Charts were available for only 45 percent of this sample. A documentation form 695-R was found in 45 percent of the charts reviewed, and 33 percent of the charts documented that a referral to a back class had been made. Only 15 percent of the charts contained documentation that the red-flag conditions had been checked.

Availability of records and compliance with the above metrics varied significantly across clinics and TMCs. Availability of medical records varied from 11 to 88 percent among MTF clinics, whereas the TMCs were more consistent, with about 50 percent of records available. TMCs also performed better than MTF clinics in rates of use of form 695-R, with 44 to 95 percent of TMC charts containing the form compared with 29 to 63 percent for the MTF clinics. TMCs also had higher rates of documented referrals to back classes. Documentation of red-flag conditions was low across all TMCs and MTF clinics, ranging from 6 to 26 percent.

Reported Effects on Clinical Practices

There was a general consensus among the Site A staff that use of the guideline had resulted in providers placing more emphasis on patient self-care, but it was uncertain whether this emphasis had any effect on other practices. Some providers perceived there was a decrease in the number of referrals to PT. There was a reported increase in MRIs for low back pain patients, but it was not necessarily attributable to the guideline. On the other hand, orthopedics expressed continued concerns about inappropriate referrals and diagnostic tests for patients with low back pain. The MTF was not yet systematically monitoring referral patterns for low back pain over time, which would be needed to assess the validity of these perceptions.

Implementation of the guideline reportedly had changed practices in the ER. Before the guideline, ER staff would attempt to manage low back pain patients on a continuous basis. By the time of our final visit, the ER staff was sending patients presenting with low back pain directly to their primary care provider after triaging for red flags and providing immediate care needs.

Conclusions

Site A approached implementation of the low back pain guideline with enthusiasm and with a strategy that emphasized patient education especially suited to a high volume and multiple-clinic setting. Initial resistance to the guideline was minimal (with some exceptions), and staff who have used it and its supporting toolkit items found it both efficient and useful.

This MTF was partially successful in its goal of emphasizing patient education. A patient referral system was put in place, and patient accessibility and referrals to back classes reportedly increased. But the early momentum proved difficult to maintain in the light of conflicting priorities, frequent deployments, and difficulties in maintaining communications among highly decentralized staff in multiple TMCs and clinics. Use of new practices was uneven and remained relatively low especially with respect to documentation of red-flag conditions. Given this situation of limited new actions, providers understandably doubt that many changes have been made in care for low back pain patients.

According to the assessment of the implementation team, the low back pain guideline was only partially implemented. The team is well aware that institutionalization of the low back pain guideline will require (1) filling the gap in guideline leadership that has slowed down implementation progress, (2) integrating training on guidelines into hospital orientation activities and possibly provider credentialing, and (3) using metrics more aggressively to monitor progress and provide feedback to clinics and individual physicians. These tasks will be a challenge because one-half of the implementation team was due to rotate during the summer of 2000. Still, the staff report having learned many lessons working on the implementation of the low back pain guideline that will enhance their ability to implement future guidelines.

SITE B

Overview of the Site Visit

The presumption at Site B was that implementation of the low back pain guideline would not affect patient outcomes because the site was already providing proper care. Thus, implementation of the low back pain guideline was given low priority at the MTF throughout the demonstration. It was formally limited to the TMCs and was hampered there by high staff turnover, limited provider education, and low provider buy-in. Implementation in the other clinics, including family practice, internal medicine, ER, and occupational health, was left to individual providers. Most providers at the MTF reported the care they provide is consistent with the guideline even if they do not use form 695-R or otherwise document the care in the chart.

The Organizational Context

Staff identified three main factors that constrained implementation of the low back pain guideline at Site B. First, unlike most other posts, this site houses a group of brigades and companies with different structures, rather than a single division. The post commander has little control over these units, except for training. In particular, medics and PAs belong to the various units, and the MTF does not have the authority to require them to use specified practices.

A second factor is that higher-priority requests took precedence over implementation of the low back pain guideline. Such items include responding to deficiencies identified in accreditation reviews, implementing anthrax vaccination that required direct reporting to the Surgeon General, a focus on pregnancy (reportedly one-half of female soldiers at the post are pregnant), and implementing TRICARE Senior Prime. They were also more concerned with medics' readiness (because units deploy to Bosnia and elsewhere) than about the low back pain guideline.

A third constraint was high staff turnover and richness of assets in some areas. High staff turnover made it difficult to educate incoming staff. With a depth of PT and chiropractic resources, there was little incentive to economize by reducing referrals to these services, regardless of whether or not the referrals were appropriate.

Attitudes Toward the Low Back Pain Guideline

Because the leadership at the MTF did not perceive there was a problem with treatment of low back pain, they believed that implementation of the guideline would have no effect on patient care and outcomes. Providers also appeared to have little concern regarding the need to appropriately document the care they provided by using form 695-R or other methods. In addition, providers reported they found the guideline was difficult to use, and that its use did not allow for patients with multiple complaints. There was also resistance to working with the guideline until it was fully automated and integrated into the clinical information system.

Implementation Activities

Implementation Strategy. The overall implementation strategy of Site B did not change from the action plan formulated at the kickoff conference. This strategy was to formally implement the low back pain guideline exclusively for care for active duty personnel, with the goal of improving the timeliness of MEB evaluations. This emphasis led to a focus on use of the guideline at the TMCs. Use of the guideline was optional for the family practice clinic, and the internal medicine clinic and the ER were not expected to use it. Finally, the MEDCOM 695-R form was to be used in the occupational health clinic, and a preventive emphasis was undertaken in an already planned primary prevention effort via injury surveillance. No progress was made on the latter two efforts because of turnover of key staff.

Implementation Team. By the end of the demonstration, the implementation team had 14 members, representing the clinical support division (1), internal medicine (2), family practice (2), troop medical (6), and PT (1), in addition to the champion and the facilitator/point of contact. Quality management personnel were never represented on the team. A significant change from earlier was the replacement of the low back pain champion, a senior officer, by a junior officer who was a young family practice physician who had recently completed his residency. He reported that he was not clear on what his role was, and he did not appear to know the details of the low back pain guideline. The full implementation team met as a group only three times following the kickoff conference, and there were no meetings in the last six months of the demonstration. The lack of cohesion in the implementation team and the low priority given to implementation of the guideline were underlined by the fact that only one-half of the team members participated in the final site visit. Reasons given for absences included permanent change of duty station rotations, other meeting commitments, or simply they were "too busy."

Provider and Ancillary Staff Education. Providers were given initial education on the low back pain guideline in early 1999, soon after the implementation kickoff conference. Reeducation on the guideline was given to providers in the internal medicine and family practice clinics at their respective December 1999 quality improvement meetings, which also covered the asthma and diabetes guidelines. About 20 minutes were dedicated to the low back pain guideline. The MTF staff estimated that 60 percent of providers at the family practice clinic and 80 percent of providers in the internal medicine clinic had been introduced to the low back pain guideline. The CME video was not used in the training sessions. In addition, providers were not aware that CME credits were available for education on the low back pain practice guideline.

About 60 percent of the TMC providers were estimated to have received some training on the guideline. The low back pain champion also had responsibility to provide monthly reviews and reminders regarding the low back pain guideline at TMC staff meetings, although the new champion gave no indication that he had followed through on this function.

Knowledge of the guideline by some providers appeared to remain superficial. For instance, two PAs interviewed at a TMC said they were familiar with the guideline, but they were unaware that their practice of frequently prescribing muscle relaxants was not recommended by the guideline.

Administrative Procedures. Most of the changes in administrative procedures in response to the low back pain guideline were made at the TMCs, reflecting Site B's implementation strategy. The documentation form 695-R was intended to be used at the TMCs. Medics had been instructed to have patients fill out the form and to place it in the patient's chart or have it available for the providers. Some providers resisted use of the form, calling it "paper pushing" and not useful. No compliance audit of the use of form 695-R was conducted, but PT staff estimated that the form was present in the chart for about 50 percent of the low back pain patients they saw. Chiropractors placed this estimate at 60 to 70 percent.

No procedural changes in support of the implementation of the low back pain guideline were made in either the family practice clinic or the internal medicine clinic. Neither clinic decided to use form 695-R in the processing of low back pain patients, and none of the individual providers interviewed from these clinics used it either. Providers also did not use the standardized profile, even though the MTF staff had identified "a large variance in temporary profiles" as an issue (as documented in our three-month site visit report).

At the time of our first site visit, the MTF had only one physical therapist, and hence, referrals to PT were discouraged. Most referrals were made to the two chiropractors participating in the Army chiropractic demonstration. By the time of our last visit, four physical therapists had arrived at the MTF, and PT referrals were encouraged. The PT staff estimated that most referrals they received were appropriate. Since the chiropractic demonstration ended, chiropractors have been integrated with PT. At the TMCs, the protocol was that patients with mechanical low back pain should be referred to PT before they are sent to orthopedics.

The orthopedics clinic at the MTF is the gatekeeper for MRI referrals and for care of chronic low back pain. This clinic either refers patients out for surgery (the site does not have a neurosurgery capability) or writes a permanent profile that limits the functions an active duty person can perform. Representatives of the orthopedics clinic estimate they approve about 20 to 25 percent of requests for MRIs. They also report a high incidence of inappropriate referrals, which were contributing to a two-week backlog for the clinic.

As of the final site visit, Site B had not changed its coding of visits to use only 724.2 as the ICD-9 diagnostic code for low back pain. Several diagnostic codes continued to be used in addition to 724.2, including 724.1, 724.5, and 724.6.

Patient Education. Patient education for low back pain is conducted individually at the discretion of providers and medics at each clinic. In general, providers use the MEDCOM patient education brochure, and medics give a copy of the brochure to patients during the visit screening. The brochure is also available in the waiting room for patients to take with them. None of the TMCs or clinics uses the patient education video. One TMC designated a medic to conduct patient education, and he sees about 25 to 30 percent of the cases.

Back classes are given at the post's wellness center. However, MTF and TMC providers do not refer active duty patients to the wellness center because the center is seen as serving primarily family members.

Table B.2 presents feedback on the toolkits provided to Site B MTFs.

Metrics and Monitoring

Site B has monitored two metrics:

- number of visits for low back pain per type of patients, using ADS
- number and disposition of MEBs.

Table B.2

Site B Assessment of Toolkit Items

Tool	Feedback from the Site
Video for CME	Not used. No comments.
MEDCOM documentation form 695-R	No specific comments by primary care providers; orthopedists liked it. General comments that the form was good to collect data and saves the provider time. Suggestion to add a diagram in the patient portion of the form to show location of the pain.
Patient education video	Not used. No comments.
Patient education brochure	Liked by most who commented.
Key elements cards	Providers said pocket card was nice for PAs to have as a reminder.
Standardized profile	Not used. No comments.
Additional toolkit items	None suggested.

About 54 percent of outpatient visits for low back pain were for active duty personnel. Between calendar years 1998 and 1999, the number of low back pain visits increased 40 percent for active duty personnel and 27 percent for non–active duty individuals. Several reasons were suggested for the increases. One was a change in TMC practice that now requires patients with low back pain to be seen by a PA. Other reasons include variations in the number of troops stationed at the post due to deployments and consolidation of TMCs into just three locations. However, these reasons do not explain the observed increases in visits for non–active duty patients. One reason pertaining to the two groups may simply be improved tracking of visits as ADS reporting increased.

The number of MEB referrals remained stable between FY 1998 and FY 1999, but it was projected to increase by 70 percent in FY 2000 based on data for the first five months of the year. Speculations were that a forthcoming deployment of troops to Bosnia accounted for this increase. In excess of 80 percent of soldiers going though the MEB process were found unfit for military service.

Site B had planned to track two additional metrics: number of referrals for MRIs and number of temporary profiles by unit. Both of these efforts were discontinued because of problems with data completeness. Because CHCS cannot track referrals for MRIs made off-post, incomplete data would underestimate actual rates of MRI referrals. For temporary profiles, the military units' operational sergeants do not accurately track and log the profiles, and different forms are used in these processes. Both issues preclude accurate measurement of these rates as well.

Reported Effects on Clinical Practices

Providers at Site B believe that the low back pain guideline had no effect on practices or patient outcomes because they believe that most providers at the TMCs were already providing effective conservative treatment. These views tend not to be supported by other information collected at the site visit. Providers believe there is a fair amount of provider shopping by low back pain patients, which suggests a lack of standardization of practices among providers on the post. At the same time, patients we interviewed expressed the views that providers are mistrustful about the reality of patients' pain and the patients' wish for more empathy. In addition, orthopedics clinic providers estimated that 20–30 percent of low back pain patients do not get the correct treatment. As stated by a site participant, they are "given a dose of Motrin and told to go away." The orthopedists report they still provide a lot of primary care for low back pain, in addition to the high incidence of referrals they receive, many of which are inappropriate. Thus, while no effects of the guideline on practices might have been achieved at this MTF, there is some qualitative evidence that such changes may be needed.

Conclusions

Site B limited its strategy for implementing the low back pain guideline to care for active duty personnel, and therefore, it limited interventions to its TMCs. Even on this limited scale, however, implementation of the guideline was approached with little support from the leadership and little guidance from the champion or the members of the implementation team. It has been particularly difficult to gauge the extent to which the guideline has actually been used. The MTF staff participating in the site visit consistently stated that they believe they were already practicing consistent with the guideline, and they were focused more on reporting the other priorities that compete with their ability to work on strengthening practices for low back pain patients. In the face of these statements, however, orthopedics providers report a continuing high incidence of inappropriate referrals for MRIs or for chronic care. Also, the MTF has not examined alternatives to strengthen the way it practices patient education: one-on-one at the discretion of providers and medics.

While a majority of providers in the family and internal medicine clinics reportedly have been introduced to the low back pain guideline, implementation has been left to the discretion of each provider within these clinics. Providers in these clinics tend to believe even more strongly than TMC providers that their practices already are consistent with the guideline.

In the words of one of the MTF providers, they "recognize that the MTF is a long way from implementing the guideline." However, many of the providers believe the experience they have gained, and difficulties they have encountered, in attempting to implement the low back pain guideline will eventually help in the implementation of subsequent guidelines. Given the contrasting reports we heard regarding the appropriateness of and variations in practices for low back pain care, it will be important to track trends in key measures to assess the status of practice quantitatively.

SITE C

Overview of the Site Visit

Support for formal implementation of the low back pain guideline at Site C appeared to falter between the three-month site visit and the final visit. A change in MTF command as well as in staff leading the implementation team may have contributed to shift emphasis away from implementation of the low back pain guideline to other priorities. One issue that has hampered implementation has been the continuing inability to gain support of the nursing and ancillary staff to use the documentation form 695-R when they process low back pain patients for provider visits. Although many providers have found the guideline helpful, many others said they were already delivering care as specified in the guideline. Follow-up on plans to gather information on the metrics has also lagged. As a result, it has not been possible to substantiate providers' claims that they are already following the guideline.

The Organizational Context

The MTF had a 50 percent turnover in its staff during the summer of 1999, including many in leadership positions. A new commander arrived during the demonstration. As of our final visit, the new commander had not seen the low back pain guideline and had not yet been briefed about it. Since our first site visit, deep differences had arisen among providers about the usefulness of the low back pain guideline and about the likely effectiveness of promoting patient self-care.

Attitudes Toward the Low Back Pain Guideline

Attitudes toward the low back pain guideline varied broadly among providers at Site C. At one extreme, one provider who recently graduated from a residency program had read the entire guideline and felt he had learned something. At the other extreme, an experienced provider thought the low back pain guideline was not the best choice to implement first because it is "a disease that is hard to monitor." Generally, younger physicians and consultants had a positive attitude toward the guideline. However, providers who had been in practice longer had more negative attitudes, stating that introducing the guideline did not improve care but only increased documentation requirements and other inefficiencies resulting from more time spent in meetings and duplicating work. This attitude is in sharp contrast to the results of a small pilot test of the documentation form 695-R that Site C had conducted at a TMC, which concluded that the form was easy to follow and allowed the TMC to process clients faster.

Implementation Activities

Implementation Strategy. The overall strategy of Site C for implementation of the low back pain guideline had not changed since our first site visit. Their strategy was to implement all components of the guideline in all clinics and TMCs for both active duty and other patients. Documentation form 695-R was seen as the primary vehicle through which compliance with the guideline would be achieved. Monitoring of selected key metrics, using ADS data and review of medical records, would permit them to assess progress and provide feedback to providers on potential issues or needed improvements.

Implementation Team. Except for loss of its original facilitator, the implementation team had remained the same since our first visit. The facilitator left because of rotation to a new assignment. The team consisted of two representatives from quality management, a pharmacist, the head nurse, a physical therapist, a sports medicine physician, nursing staff, and ancillary staff. The team reportedly meets monthly as part of a broader effort to implement pathways at the MTF. Team participants reported that a civilian member of the staff had carried out the bulk of the work to implement the guideline.

Nine of the team members met with us during our last site visit. The low back pain guideline champion, who has been a strong advocate for the guideline, was on travel duty at the time of the visit. Also, the chief of ER and a representative from occupational health who were on the implementation team at our first visit were not present during our second visit.

Provider and Ancillary Staff Education. One-half of the medical providers at the MTF have turned over since the kickoff conference for the low back pain guideline demonstration, creating a large workload for efforts to educate newcomers on the low back pain guideline. The new arrivals came from both military and civilian residencies. They were educated on the low back pain guideline as part of a three-hour session integrated into a two-day orientation to the MTF held in August of 1999.

By contrast, ancillary staff did not receive formal orientation to the low back pain guideline but were introduced to it only through some on-the-job training. This lack of attention to ancillary staff training may have contributed to their widespread unwillingness to integrate use of documentation form 695-R within their routine processing of patients.

Administrative Processes. Use of documentation form 695-R was to be the primary vehicle through which the low back pain practice guideline would be followed and documented at the MTF. Although use of the form increased from 4 to 20 percent of patients between our first and second visits (based on chart audits), use remained low. According to providers participating in the site visit, at least part of this problem was because the form was not inserted into the patient chart or otherwise readily available to them, which frustrated those providers who wanted to use the form to document care. Unavailability of forms was widely attributed to lack of cooperation by the nursing and ancillary staff. Several reasons were given for this lack of cooperation:

- Use of the form is additional work.
- Patient confidentiality cannot be protected given lack of space or physical layout.
- The mind-set among nursing and ancillary staff was that the form is the provider's responsibility.
- Nursing and ancillary staff were overworked because of the low ratio of 0.8 support staff to provider staff.
- Perceptions by nursing and ancillary staff were that the form was a test form and not required.
- Patients resisted repeatedly filling out the form at every visit.
- There were language problems with patients who do not speak English well.

The net effect of these issues was that no permanent changes in administrative procedures were implemented. There was a sense that providers did not feel comfortable placing demands on the ancillary staff, who they knew were overworked, and that command did not see the low back pain guideline as a priority. But some providers have succeeded in making the process work for them. At least one provider reported having no problem with ancillary staff in requiring that the form be filled out by the patients and available with the chart during examination. Also, there were perceptions that contract providers were using the form more frequently because it helped them see more patients and, since they had higher ratios of support to provider staff, ancillary staff had time to process the forms.

No new procedures were put in place to increase referrals to back classes. Such referrals remain at the discretion of the physician. Similarly, there are no procedures to follow up on patients who fail to attend a back class after making an appointment.

The implementation team raised three additional procedural issues. The first concerned placement of the documentation form 695-R in the patient chart. It was pointed out that Army regulations require that only form SF-600 may be filed in chronological order in the chart. All other forms have to been placed at the end or on the left side. Providers expressed frustration with lack of standardization in filing the form and having to look for it.

Second, Site C had difficulties standardizing use of MEDCOM's designated unique ICD-9 code on the ADS form because of staff turnover and lack of training. Downtime on the ADS and backlogs for completing the ADS form added to the problem of timely documentation and limited the usefulness of the ADS for monitoring progress in implementation of the guideline. Delays in completion of the "bubble" sheet occurred because of inadequate support staff and the tendency of providers to give priority to spending their time on treatment of patients rather than completing the ADS sheets.

Finally, the MTF staff continued to view use of the documentation form 695-R for repeat visits as a burden that takes away valuable clinical interactive time between provider and patients.

Patient Education. Three basic vehicles are used at Site C to provide education for low back pain patients: back class, one-on-one education by providers, and the MEDCOM patient education brochures. Primary care providers refer patients to back class at their individual discretion. Classes are held every other Tuesday. On average, about 12 patients attend each class, most of whom reportedly have attended the class previously. Perceptions are that attendance at back class has not increased since the low back pain guideline was introduced. Patients who are referred are not tracked, although primary care providers say they would welcome feedback on patients who did not show up for the class.

The MEDCOM brochures are available at the clinics, and providers say they use the brochure in talking to their patients. It reportedly allows providers to explain appropriate exercises and preventive behavior faster to the patient. However, a physical therapist conducted a survey of low back pain patients referred to him and found that none of the patients had received or seen any educational material for low back pain. Thus, there is substantial uncertainty regarding the extent to which patient education is being provided in the primary care clinics.

The patient education video was not used at Site C because of an insufficient supply of video players to show the video regularly, and most staff thought they had only one tape available. It turned out that several copies had been received, but they had not been distributed. Alternatively, closed circuit television could be used for this purpose, and this possibility is being considered.

Table B.3 presents feedback on the toolkits provided to Site C MTFs.

Metrics and Monitoring

The original plans by Site C for monitoring progress in guideline implementation have been hampered by time constraints, breakdowns in the ADS, inaccurate and untimely ADS coding, and difficulties in accessing the CHCS data. By the time of our final visit, Site C had focused on measuring two metrics:

- presence of documentation form 695-R in medical charts
- number of MRIs ordered.

Table B.3

Site C Assessment of Toolkit Items

Tool	Feedback from the Site
Video for CME	No feedback provided.
MEDCOM documentation form 695-R	Positive comments about the original form included the following: helps efficiency by seeing patients faster, a useful reminder of red-flag conditions, the pain scale is useful to assess progress, helps process new Army recruits efficiently to make a decision whether to continue training or release from service. Most staff thought the form should be filled out only at the first visit. They also felt the form was not useful for patients presenting with multiple problems.
Patient education video	No feedback provided. Few staff had seen it.
Patient education brochure	Generally liked, but some felt it did not do much good with their patients. It should include an explanation to patients of why taking an X ray was not indicated.
Key elements card	Both cards are useful as reminders, most particularly for young providers and those who do not see many low back pain patients.
Standardized profile	No feedback provided. Used at the discretion of the provider.

As noted above, the presence of form 695-R in charts had increased from 4 to 20 percent between our two site visits to the MTF. No other information (e.g., documentation of red flags) was retrieved from the medical records. The number of MRIs increased from an average of 51 to 75 annually. The previous commander established a directive to use CT scans instead of MRIs because the latter have to be done off-post at additional cost. According to staff, the increase in MRIs might be caused by the influx of new physicians, who might have been less aware of the command directive. All MRI referrals have to be approved by the chief of the clinic and cleared by the chief of orthopedics. There is no information on the appropriateness of these referrals.

One provider performed an analysis of the length of time that active duty patients with low back pain had been in treatment over the period of October 1998 to November 1999. About 56 percent of patients were in treatment for one month or less and an additional 16 percent were in treatment for one to two months. Only 7 percent of patients had been in treatment for six months or more.

Reported Effects on Clinical Practices

As stated above, the low back pain guideline may have contributed to an increase in MRIs, although data were not available to assess the appropriateness of those referrals. According to perceptions of the implementation team and staff interviewed, the guideline has had no effect on patterns of referrals to PT, chiropractors, CT scans, or MEB. They also report that some providers continue to prescribe muscle relaxants for low back pain patients, which the guideline specifically identifies as inappropriate. While most providers reported their practices had not changed since introduction of the guideline, a few thought otherwise. More data are needed to assess the extent to which these perceptions are accurate.

Representatives of the orthopedic department stated there was a lack of adherence to the low back pain guideline with regard to specialty referrals, most particularly by physician assistants. They estimated that 80 percent of referrals for orthopedic diagnostic studies were inappropriate, contributing to a four to six week backlog in orthopedics. They believe there is a need for more provider education on performing a proper physical examination for low back pain patients.

The handling of patients referred to chiropractors has changed since the introduction of the guideline. The chiropractors now send all low back pain patients back to primary care providers after a six-week period of treatment. There was discussion regarding whether the number of treatment sessions might be a better yardstick to guide this decision than length of time.

Conclusions

After an active start in implementation of the low back pain guideline at Site C, interventions to change practices declined and became more sporadic. By the time of our last site visit, most actions appeared to be left to the discretion of individual providers, with little proactive organizational support to assist them. The MTF's implementation strategy relied primarily on the integration of documentation form 695-R into procedures for processing low back pain patients during clinic visits, and on having this form available to the provider during treatment. Its success depended on the cooperation of the nursing and ancillary staff. When these staff refused to cooperate in this task, no formal action was taken by the MTF management to resolve the problem. As a result, implementation of the guideline fell by default to providers and to one civilian member of the implementation team who had neither the time nor authority to address this issue. Multiple issues contributed to making the nursing and ancillary staff unwilling to cooperate, including severe workloads due to low ratios of support to provider staff and lack of formal training of these staff in the purpose of the guideline and the documentation form. Providers state that in practice they follow the guideline even if they do not fully document it, but at this point there are no data to confirm or refute these perceptions.

A set of specific management and administrative issues also appear to have contributed to loss of momentum in implementing the low back pain guideline at Site C. First, staffing constraints, as reflected in low ratios of support to provider staff, made it difficult to add new tasks to the workload of nursing and ancillary staff. Second, changes in MTF command during the demonstration period appear to have relegated guideline implementation to a lower priority. Third, there were questions regarding whether or not to use the documentation form 695-R for repeat visits and where the form was to be filed within the medical chart. Finally, information system issues impaired the ability to develop metrics to monitor progress in changing clinical practices, including periodic difficulties with reliability of the ADS and barriers to making changes in coding for low back pain.

SITE D

Overview of the Site Visit

Site D has used the low back pain guideline primarily to modify and coordinate the way it treats chronic low back pain cases. The acute care portion of the guideline was introduced in all clinics and the consolidated troop medical clinic (CTMC), giving physicians discretion about whether to use it and the documentation form 695-R. Emphasis was placed on providing a minimum of three to four weeks of conservative treatment before referring for specialist treatment. To reduce inappropriate specialty referrals for low back pain patients, the physical medicine and rehabilitation clinic was designated as gatekeeper for referrals to specialist care and to serve as consultant to primary care physicians for management of these patients. Site D monitored trends on a number of relevant metrics using ADS and CHCS data.

The Organizational Context

The hospital at Site D has undergone major changes in leadership and the way it delivers health care. The new paradigm being put in place emphasizes primary care and preventive services. At the same time the MTF is deploying the Clinical Integrated Workplace (CIW) information system, which is expected to eventually provide electronic access to guidelines and forms, and ease documentation of care. The MTF has introduced about 30 clinical pathways or guidelines for inpatient care. While use of guidelines in tertiary care has been widely accepted at Site D, their use for primary care has met resistance.

All new TRICARE enrollees at Site D are assigned to a clinic and physician. They also receive a 45-minute patient assessment at their first visit and are given a self-care booklet. As their health conditions may indicate, patients are referred to relevant classes, including back classes.

As a medical center, the MTF has a large number of specialties that are relevant to the care of low back pain. These include neurology, anesthesiology, sports/physical medicine, osteopathy, rheumatology, orthopedics, psychology, and neurosurgery. It has been difficult to coordinate treatment for a given low back pain patient among these specialties.

Attitudes Toward the Low Back Pain Guideline

Although the MTF leadership at Site D has supported implementation of the low back pain guideline, the implementation team reports that there is "no enthusiasm" among staff to do so. Resistance to use the guideline appears to be stronger among physicians than among PAs and general medical officers. Physicians reportedly feel the guideline is not theirs, and they would have liked more of a say regarding its contents. Perceptions that implementation of the guideline might generate more work are also contributing to their reluctance to change practices. Another reason is doubt that there will be useful outcomes: "Use of the guideline will not change at-risk patient's behavior and will put more soldiers on profile." The guideline is viewed as not being useful for managing Army trainees with low back pain, where the focus is on identification of trainees who should be discharged. About 4 to 5 percent of the trainees assigned to this post already have a profile (specified limitation of function) for low back pain at arrival.

Implementation Activities

Implementation Strategy. Implementation of the portion of the guideline addressing management of acute low back pain focused on the CTMC, although all clinics were introduced to the guideline and its recommendation that initial low back pain patients be treated conservatively for at least three to four weeks. Emphasis was also placed on developing an electronic version of documentation form 695-R. Automation of the documentation form was seen as a key to eventual provider buy-in at the CTMC, as well as in the MTF primary care clinics. The implementation team has encouraged the ER to use the low back pain guideline, but the ER staff continue to be unwilling to implement the guideline.

Concerns about inappropriate low back pain referrals to specialties, especially neurosurgery, and lack of standardization of care led Site D to designate the physical medicine and rehabilitation clinic as the gatekeeper for assessment and coordination of specialty referrals and chronic low back pain cases. In that role, the physical medicine and rehabilitation clinic initiated a program of weekly meetings with representatives of various specialties to coordinate the treatment of complex cases involving multiple specialties.

Implementation Team. Site D started with an 18-member implementation team. The team was soon reduced to 7 members including representation from UM, QM, physical medicine, occupational health, family practice, PT, and the CTMC. This reduced team met a couple of times early in the demonstration and then stopped meeting for several months. The team was reconstituted about four months prior to our March 2000 visit. It initially met bimonthly and, at the time of our final visit, was meeting monthly. The champion and the facilitator have performed the majority of the implementation work.

The champion and facilitator introduced the guideline one-on-one to each member of the team, and the facilitator developed the automated version of form 695-R. He devoted to this task about 45 percent of his time for several months.

Provider and Ancillary Education. When Site D began implementing the low back pain guideline, the guideline champion and the chief of physical medicine used the CME videotape to train providers on the guideline at each clinic. However, CME credits were not given to the providers. New interns were also educated on the guideline. Ancillary staff were not formally trained on the guideline. After the educational activities, the laminated pocket cards with the guideline "key elements" were distributed to the providers.

Education on practice guidelines was not integrated into the orientation program for new MTF staff, although the implementation team thought it should be. In addition, the implementation team recognized a need for ongoing education and refreshers for existing staff. However, no procedures to do so had been established as of the date of our final visit.

Administrative Procedures. Administrative procedures for processing low back pain patients differ between the CTMC and the primary care clinics at the hospital. At the CTMC, the documentation form 695-R is given to the low back pain patients at the check-in desk. Reportedly, 80 to 90 percent of these patients entered the screening rooms with the form. The form is filled out at every encounter because some providers (mostly PAs and general medical officers) monitor patients' progress on the pain scale. Yet the team reports that ensuring consistency in this process remains difficult, and there has been a reported "erosion" over time in the use of form 695-R. Filling out the patient portion of the form takes time, lengthening the visit process. In addition, medics rotate every two weeks, and new medics must constantly be trained in the procedures.

To facilitate processing of patients and minimize paperwork, an automated form 695-R was developed and integrated into the CIW system. The use of this form was tested first at the CTMC. The intent was for the medics to work with the patients in the screening room to fill out the patient portion of the form. That information and the provider portion of the form are available on the provider's computer screen, and the provider completes the form online. Although Site D has received the revised 695-R form, it has not yet been distributed for use or had its revisions incorporated into the form in the CIW system.

Low back pain patients are treated at the CTMC for a period of three to four weeks. If the condition persists after that time, they are referred to PT (the MTF has three physical therapists) or for manipulation for one week or so. If the condition persists after this treatment, patients are referred to the physical medicine clinic for assessment and either referral to the appropriate specialist(s) or permanent profiling. Treatment of difficult cases involving multiple specialists is coordinated in weekly meetings chaired by a physical medicine provider. These meetings are a new mechanism established as part of the guideline implementation strategy.

At the clinics, implementation of the low back pain guideline (and use of documentation form 695-R) was left to the physicians' discretion. It is a hit and miss process. No formal procedure has been put in place other than for patients whose conditions persist beyond six weeks and who are to be referred to the physical medicine clinic for assessment and appropriate referral(s) or profiling.

Site D has not yet fully adopted the unique ICD-9 code for low back pain (724.2) that was established by MEDCOM, although there has been an increase in the use of this code. Its providers continue to use primarily code 724.5, as well as 724.1, 724.7, 724.8, and 724.9.

Patient Education. Patient education is handled differently at the CTMC and at the family practice clinic. At the CTMC, low back pain patients are referred to the wellness center for back classes at the first encounter. The referral is handled as a consult via CHCS. The patient education pamphlets are available in the clinic waiting room, but not in the examination rooms. At the family practice clinic, providers perform the patient education themselves. Pamphlets are available in the examination room.

Table B.4 presents feedback on the toolkits provided to Site D MTFs.

Metrics and Monitoring

Site D took a strong initiative in monitoring and has been tracking a number of metrics for low back pain patients via ADS and CHCS. In addition, a sample of charts at the CTMC and ER were reviewed to assess use of the 695-R form, documentation of red-flag conditions,

Table B.4

Site D Assessment of Toolkit Items

Tool	Feedback from the Site
Video for CME	No comments.
MEDCOM documentation form 695-R	Some providers find the form useful as a reminder. Those who use it find it is efficient for documenting treatment, and some look at changes from visit to visit on the pain scale. Patients find it time consuming to fill out the form and some have difficulty doing it. Some patients complain about having to fill it out at every visit. A lower level of reading is needed, and the form should be available in several languages.
Patient education video	Used in the wellness center only. No comments.
Patient education brochure	No comments.
Key elements cards	No comments.
Standardized profiles	No comments.
Additional toolkit items	None suggested.

presence of treatment plans, referrals, and co-morbidity factors. The service activity measures being tracked include

- number of encounters and patients, by month, clinic, type of patient, and type of appointment (i.e., scheduled appointment, walk-in, or sick call)
- dispositions of visits (i.e., inpatient admission, immediate referrals, received profile, remain at quarters, and return without leave)
- frequency of encounters
- frequency of visits to PT
- pattern of use of ancillary services and drugs per provider.

Thus far, trends in encounters have been monitored from January through December 1999. Overall, the total number of encounters remained relatively constant from month to month, but there was a change in the distribution of encounters across clinics. The physical medicine clinic began functioning as the gatekeeper for chronic cases in the spring, and about 20 percent of all encounters for low back pain began to be diverted to it. An examination of trends over the following six months suggests that the CTMC has been the largest beneficiary of this shift. Its share of total encounters declined from 40 percent or greater to 30 percent immediately after the shift, and subsequently declined to about 25 percent by the end of the year. The number of orthopedics encounters also declined sharply, while encounters in neurosurgery declined slightly and then climbed back to their earlier numbers. The number of encounters at the ER has remained constant.

The Site D implementation team reported service activity for low back pain patients for clinic visits, PT, ancillary services, and prescription medications, although trends on how utilization changed with introduction of the guideline were not reported. Of patients who have had more than one encounter for low back pain, two out of three had two encounters and another 20 percent had three encounters. Less than two percent of low back pain patients had seven or more encounters excluding PT. Two out of three patients who were referred to PT went for four or fewer sessions. However, about 10 percent of referred patients receive 20 or more PT sessions with some as many as 45 sessions. There are large variations among primary care providers in their pattern of referrals to ancillary services (CT scan and MRI) and in the drugs they prescribe (Valium, Robaxin, Flexeril). The greatest variation is in the use of Flexeril, with some providers preferring using other drugs (e.g., Robaxin) and others using it exclusively of any others.

During the calendar year 1999, there was a shift in the distribution of dispositions for active duty personnel with low back pain. The patients with profiles declined from nearly one-half of the dispositions to less than 25 percent, while returns without leave increased. Other dispositions remained relatively constant, ranging between 5 and 13 percent for immediate referrals and between 6 and 10 percent for assignment to quarters. On average, there was one inpatient admission due to low back pain per month for active duty personnel. Site D also keeps track of its patients on permanent profiles. The number of low back pain patients increased from 42 in 1998 to 73 in 1999. Typically, up to 50 percent of these patients end up referred to MEB.

The chart review performed at the CTMC in March 1999 showed that form 695-R was present in a relatively high portion of the medical charts, but there was a low rate of documentation that the provider had checked the patient for red-flag conditions. About 300 CTMC patients were drawn as the sample. Charts were available for only 60 patients, of which 27 were actually reviewed. For these 27 patients *with* a 695-R form, 67 percent were appropriately coded as having low back pain, 19 percent had documentation that the red flags had been checked, and 56 percent had a profile in the chart.

Appropriateness of referrals was not being monitored as of the time of our final site visit. PT staff estimated that 5 percent of the referrals they received were inappropriate, while neurosurgery staff estimated that 10 percent of the referrals they received were inappropriate.

Reported Effects on Clinical Practices

In general, the Site D staff perceived that the low back pain guideline had little, if any, effect on clinical practices for care of acute low back pain. Staff believed conservative care was already being provided to acute low back pain patients, and the emphasis continued to be placed on getting soldiers back to training. Some staff indicated, however, that the low back pain guideline contributed to the decline in the relative number of profiles written and to the increase in the number of referrals to MEB.

Some staff in the family practice clinic indicated that staff at that clinic had not been familiar with low back pain treatment, and the guideline education and the key element cards they received had been helpful. Also, PT staff reported an increase in PT referrals.

Clinical practice for chronic cases has changed with the designation of a gatekeeper for referrals and coordinator for complicated cases. According to the team members, "This has helped standardize the treatment of chronic care cases." Reportedly, patients feel they are not bounced around the hospital under this new arrangement. Establishment of the gatekeeper function is also credited with reducing the backlog in neurosurgery from three months to two weeks.

Conclusions

Site D is seeking to integrate the implementation of the low back pain guideline into the hospital's new paradigm of care that places more emphasis on primary care and prevention. Having the perception that conservative treatment was already being provided for acute low back pain cases, the MTF focused initially on the portion of the guideline addressing management of chronic cases. An emphasis was placed on designating one clinic as the gatekeeper to resolve existing difficulties with inappropriate referrals of low back pain patients to neurosurgery and inadequate coordination with the numerous relevant specialties available at the medical center. At the same time, the MTF sought to formally implement use of the guideline in its CTMC and other primary care clinics. There was substantial initial buy-in for the guideline recommendations, but turnover and other pressures reportedly led to a decline in compliance over time.

MTF leadership at Site D believes that full compliance with the low back pain guideline, and eventually any guideline for primary care, cannot occur without increasing electronic applications related to the guideline, especially online documentation of care. To this end, the MTF developed its own computerized algorithm for management of low back pain that follows the guideline in steps and allows online checks of the examinations performed and treatment provided. This approach was being tested at the CTMC at the time of our final visit. An important issue, which is a chronic problem in MTFs, is that this automated system was created by one entrepreneurial, computer savvy military person, who left in the summer rotations, and his computer skills will be difficult to replicate. This issue speaks to the need for systemwide applications to institutionalize such systems.

Appendix C

MULTIVARIATE ANALYSES OF LOW BACK PAIN METRICS

To test for effects of the introduction of the DoD/VA low back pain guideline on service utilization and prescription patterns, we fit a series of regression models to predict each of the six measures of guideline effects during the treatment of acute low back pain. We calculated the following measures for activity within six weeks of the initial low back pain encounter:

- whether a patient was referred to PT
- the number of follow-up primary care visits
- whether a patient was referred to specialty care
- whether a patient was prescribed muscle relaxants
- whether a patient was prescribed narcotics
- whether an NSAID prescription was for a high-cost NSAID.

The unit of analysis for the first five measures was the episode of care, so there was one record in the data file used for each episode of care with variables for the five measures. As described in Chapter Two, this study was limited to episodes of low back pain care for active duty Army personnel. The variables for PT referrals, specialty referrals, muscle relaxant prescriptions, and narcotic prescriptions were dichotomous variables (equal to one if one of these events had occurred). For these measures, we used logistic regression models to test the size and statistical significance of effects.

The variable for follow-up primary care visits was a count of the number of visits that occurred during an episode of care. For this measure, we estimated an ordered logit regression model. Most patients had zero or one follow-up primary care visit within six weeks of the initial low back pain encounter, and only 5 percent had two or more visits. Therefore, we defined a three-level outcome variable (0, 1, 2+ visits) for the ordered logit model to test for a guideline effect.

The unit of analysis for the use of high-cost NSAIDs was the NSAID prescription, and the sample was all NSAID prescriptions for episodes of care included in the study. A dichotomous variable was set equal to one if the NSAID was a high-cost one. We used a logistic regression model to test effects for this measure.

The predictor variables in the models included dummy variables for each quarter (with quarter 2 omitted as the referent variable), a dummy variable for the demonstration site, and variables to control for patient characteristics. Using SIDPERS data, we controlled for the patient characteristics of gender, rank (officer versus enlisted), and age categories. The referent age category in our models was 18–29 years, and the other two categories were 30–39 years and 40 years or older. We collapsed the two control groups into one group for all analyses because we found no difference in trends between them.

Guideline effects were measured using interaction terms of the demonstration site by each of the three quarter dummy variables for the demonstration period (the third through fifth quarters). The coefficient on each quarter variable estimated the difference in a measure between demonstration and control sites relative to the baseline period, i.e., the effects of the demonstration.

In logistic regression models, the magnitude of effect for a unit change in a variable can be expressed as an odds ratio, which is obtained by exponentiating the variable's coefficient. An odds ratio is defined as the odds that an outcome variable will occur divided by the odds that it will not occur. An odds ratio for a predictor variable that is equal to one (equal odds) indicates that the variable has no effect on the occurrence of the outcome. An odds ratio greater than one indicates that the variable increases the probability of the outcome occurring, and an odds ratio of less than one indicates that it decreases the probability. We report here both the statistical significance of the predictor variable coefficients and the odds ratios for the models estimated for the six low back pain metrics listed above.

REFERRALS TO PT OR MANIPULATION SERVICES

The results of the logistic regression analysis for trends in referrals to PT or manipulation services are reported in Table C.1. There was little temporal trend in referral rates, as shown by the consistent coefficients and odds ratios for the quarter variables, and referral rates for demonstration and control sites were not significantly different—$p < 0.10$ on the "demo" (demonstration site) variable. The significant odds ratios for the interaction terms for demo × quarters indicate that patients in the demonstration sites were less likely to be referred to PT in the last two quarters, compared with the control sites (odds ratios of 0.7 for the fourth and fifth quarters). This result suggests that use of the guideline reduced PT referral rates for the demonstration sites. Also of interest, neither gender nor rank was a significant predictor of PT referrals, but active duty personnel older than 29 years of age were referred more frequently than the younger personnel.

FOLLOW-UP PRIMARY CARE VISITS

The results of the ordered logistic regression analysis of follow-up primary care visits for acute low back pain patients are presented in Table C.2. As discussed above, the outcome variable for this analysis was a three-level variable of 0, 1, or 2+ follow-up visits after the initial visit. The observed upward trend in control site visit rates during the last three quarters was found to be significant, as shown by the variables for quarters 4 and 5. Further, the significant interaction term for the last quarter (demo × quarter 5) and its odds ratio of 0.7 indicate that the demonstration sites had a significant reduction in frequency of follow-up visits in that quarter, compared with the control sites. Although this decline could be the start of a trend related to the use of the guideline, it would be necessary to track this measure for subsequent periods of time before attributing such an effect to the guideline. Also of interest, all the demographic characteristics of the low back pain patients had significant independent effects on the frequency of follow-up visits. Older patients and officers had fewer follow-up visits than younger enlisted patients, and females had more visits than males.

Table C.1

Logistic Regression Model of Estimated Guideline Effects on Referrals to PT or Manipulation Services Within Six Weeks of Initial Visit

Parameter	Estimated Coefficient	Standard Error	Odds Ratio
Female	–0.05	0.05	1.0
Officer	0.09	0.07	1.1
Age 30–39	0.22***	0.04	1.3
Age 40 or older	0.23**	0.06	1.3
Demo (1, 0)	–0.11+	0.06	0.9
Quarter 1	–0.18**	0.06	0.8
Quarter 3	–0.17*	0.08	0.9
Quarter 4	–0.08	0.07	0.9
Quarter 5	–0.11	0.08	0.9
Interaction terms:			
Demo × quarter 3	–0.02	0.10	1.0
Demo × quarter 4	–0.33***	0.10	0.7
Demo × quarter 5	–0.38***	0.11	0.7
Intercept	–2.14	0.09	

NOTES: + $p < 0.10$, * $p < 0.05$, ** $p < 0.01$, *** $p < 0.001$. The omitted group for the model is quarter 2, which is the baseline time period that immediately preceded the start of implementation activities by the demonstration MTFs.

REFERRALS TO SPECIALTY CARE

The results of the logistic regression analysis of trends in specialty care referrals are reported in Table C.3. This analysis was performed using three of the four demonstration sites. Site B was excluded because of its unexplained escalation in referrals of low back pain patients to orthopedics, which would confound any trends for the other facilities (see Figures 6.7 and 6.8). Overall, the demonstration sites were less likely to refer acute low back pain patients to specialty care than the control sites, as shown by the significant and low odds ratio (0.8) for the demo variable. The significant coefficients and low odds ratios for the variables for quarters 4 and 5 indicate a downward trend in control site specialty referrals during the demonstration period. None of the interaction terms for the three demonstration quarters (quarters 3 through 5) is significant and their odds ratios

Table C.2

Ordered Logit Model of Estimated Guideline Effects on Frequency of Follow-Up Primary Care Visits Within Six Weeks of Initial Visit

Parameter	Estimated Coefficient	Standard Error	Odds Ratio
Female	0.09**	0.03	1.1
Officer	–0.21***	0.05	0.8
Age 30–39	–0.44***	0.03	0.6
Age 40 or older	–0.82***	0.04	0.4
Demo (1, 0)	0.39***	0.04	1.5
Quarter 1	–0.06	0.04	0.9
Quarter 3	0.02	0.05	1.0
Quarter 4	0.10*	0.05	1.1
Quarter 5	0.15**	0.05	1.2
Interaction terms:			
Demo × quarter 3	–0.09	0.07	0.9
Demo × quarter 4	–0.06	0.07	0.9
Demo × quarter 5	–0.30***	0.07	0.7
Intercept 1	–2.73	0.06	
Intercept 2	1.59	0.06	

NOTES: + $p < 0.10$, * $p < 0.05$, ** $p < 0.01$, *** $p < 0.001$. The omitted group for the model is quarter 2, which is the baseline time period that immediately preceded the start of implementation activities by the demonstration MTFs.

are close to 1.0, thus indicating the demonstration did not affect overall specialty referrals for the three demonstration sites. Also of interest, older active duty personnel were two to four times more likely to be referred for specialty care for their acute low back pain than were younger personnel. In addition, officers were more likely then enlisted patients to be referred to specialists.

PRESCRIPTION OF MUSCLE RELAXANTS

The results of the logistic regression analysis of trends in muscle relaxant prescription are reported in Table C.4. Overall, the demonstration sites were less likely than the control sites to prescribe muscle relaxants for acute low back pain patients, as shown by the significant coefficient and low odds ratio for the demo variable. However, the interaction terms for quarters 3 and 4 (demo × quarter) reveal

Table C.3

Logistic Regression Model of Estimated Guideline Effects on Referrals to Specialty Care Within Six Weeks of Initial Visit

Parameter	Estimated Coefficient	Standard Error	Odds Ratio
Female	–0.03	0.05	1.0
Officer	0.31***	0.06	1.4
Age 30–39	0.91***	0.05	2.5
Age 40 or older	1.44***	0.06	4.4
Demo (1, 0)	–0.20***	0.06	0.8
Quarter 1	0.18**	0.06	1.2
Quarter 3	0.04	0.08	1.0
Quarter 4	–0.15+	0.08	0.9
Quarter 5	–0.23**	0.09	0.8
Interaction terms:			
Demo × quarter 3	–0.14	0.12	0.9
Demo × quarter 4	–0.09	0.12	0.9
Demo × quarter 5	0.06	0.12	1.1
Intercept	–3.06	0.09	

NOTES: + $p < 0.10$, * $p < 0.05$, ** $p < 0.01$, *** $p < 0.001$. The omitted group for the model is quarter 2, which is the baseline time period that immediately preceded the start of implementation activities by the demonstration MTFs.

that the probability of prescribing muscle relaxants increased during the demonstration for the demonstration sites, which is the opposite of the guideline recommendation. At the same time, prescription of muscle relaxants in the control sites remained relatively unchanged (i.e., the variables for quarters 3 through 5 were not statistically significant). Also of interest, active duty patients age 30–39 were more likely to be prescribed muscle relaxants than either their younger or older counterparts, and officers were less likely to be prescribed these medications.

PRESCRIPTION OF NARCOTICS

The results of the logistic regression analysis of trends in the percentage of patients prescribed narcotics are reported in Table C.5. Overall, providers at the demonstration sites were less likely than

Table C.4

Logistic Regression Model of Estimated Guideline Effects on Prescription of Muscle Relaxants Within Six Weeks of Initial Visit

Parameter	Estimated Coefficient	Standard Error	Odds Ratio
Female	0.02	0.03	1.0
Officer	–0.12**	0.04	0.9
Age 30–39	0.11***	0.03	1.1
Age 40 or older	–0.19***	0.04	0.8
Demo (1, 0)	–0.37***	0.04	0.7
Quarter 1	–0.04	0.04	1.0
Quarter 3	–0.06	0.05	0.9
Quarter 4	–0.02	0.05	1.0
Quarter 5	0.05	0.05	1.1
Interaction terms:			
Demo × quarter 3	0.14*	0.06	1.1
Demo × quarter 4	0.13*	0.06	1.1
Demo × quarter 5	–0.01	0.06	1.0
Intercept	0.27	0.07	

NOTES: + $p < 0.10$, * $p < 0.05$, ** $p < 0.01$, *** $p < 0.001$. The omitted group for the model is quarter 2, which is the baseline time period that immediately preceded the start of implementation activities by the demonstration MTFs.

those at the control sites to prescribe narcotics to acute low back pain patients, as indicated by the significant coefficient and low odds ratio for the demo variable. We found a significant downward trend for the control sites in the probability that low back pain patients would be prescribed muscle relaxants during the demonstration period (quarters 3 through 5). In addition, the trend for the demonstration sites did not differ from the control site trend, as shown by the nonsignificant coefficients on the interaction terms (demo × quarter). This finding confirms the results observed in Figure 6.12 indicating that use of the low back pain guideline was not associated with reductions in use of narcotics for acute low back pain patients. Also of interest, narcotics were more likely to be prescribed to women than to men and to patients age 30 or older (compared with those younger than age 30). Further, officers were less likely to be prescribed narcotics than enlisted personnel (odds ratio = 0.9).

Table C.5

Logistic Regression Model of Estimated Guideline Effects on Prescription of Narcotics Within Six Weeks of Initial Visit

Parameter	Estimated Coefficient	Standard Error	Odds Ratio
Female	0.35***	0.03	1.4
Officer	–0.15***	0.05	0.9
Age 30–39	0.25***	0.03	1.3
Age 40 or older	0.30***	0.04	1.4
Demo (1, 0)	–0.21***	0.04	0.8
Quarter 1	0.05	0.04	1.0
Quarter 3	–0.18***	0.05	0.8
Quarter 4	–0.16**	0.05	0.9
Quarter 5	–0.24***	0.05	0.8
Interaction terms:			
Demo × quarter 3	0.17**	0.07	1.2
Demo × quarter 4	0.05	0.07	1.1
Demo × quarter 5	0.03	0.07	1.0
Intercept	–0.55	0.06	

NOTES: + $p < 0.10$, * $p < 0.05$, ** $p < 0.01$, *** $p < 0.001$. The omitted group for the model is quarter 2, which is the baseline time period that immediately preceded the start of implementation activities by the demonstration MTFs.

PRESCRIPTION OF HIGH-COST NSAIDs

The results of the logistic regression analysis of trends in high-cost NSAID prescriptions are reported in Table C.6. We estimated this model using data for all the demonstration and control sites, including the two MTFs (one demonstration and one control) where use of high-cost NSAIDs increased over time. Figure 6.14 shows that these two MTFs substantially affected observed trends in percentages of high-cost NSAIDs during the study period. Overall, the significant coefficient and odds ratio of 2.3 for the demo variable show that providers at the demonstration sites were more likely than those at the control sites to choose a high-cost NSAID when prescribing NSAIDs for their patients. The time trend variables for the control sites during the demonstration period showed no trend in the percentages of high-cost NSAIDs prescribed in the third or fourth quarters, followed by a small but significant increase in use in the fifth quarter.

Table C.6

Logistic Regression Model of Estimated Guideline Effects on Prescription of High-Cost NSAIDs Within Six Weeks of Initial Visit

Parameter	Estimated Coefficient	Standard Error	Odds Ratio
Female	0.28***	0.05	1.3
Officer	0.11	0.07	1.1
Age 30–39	0.71***	0.05	2.0
Age 40+	1.33***	0.06	3.8
Demo (1, 0)	0.82***	0.07	2.3
Quarter 1	–0.21**	0.07	0.8
Quarter 3	0.15	0.11	1.2
Quarter 4	0.10	0.11	1.1
Quarter 5	0.23*	0.11	1.3
Interaction terms:			
Demo × quarter 3	0.04	0.12	1.0
Demo × quarter 4	0.23+	0.12	1.3
Demo × quarter 5	0.18	0.12	1.2
Intercept	–4.42	0.13	

NOTES: + $p < 0.10$, * $p < 0.05$, ** $p < 0.01$, *** $p < 0.001$. The omitted group for the model is quarter 2, which is the baseline time period that immediately preceded the start of implementation activities by the demonstration MTFs.

No significant differences were shown between the demonstration and control sites in any of the three quarters, as indicated by the nonsignificant interaction terms (demo × quarter). Thus, the introduction of the low back pain guideline did not have an observable effect on the probability that providers would use high-cost NSAIDs for low back pain patients. When the two outlier MTFs were removed from the sample, we obtained a trend of slightly decreasing use of high-cost NSAIDs, but again, no differences were found between the demonstration and control sites.

Also of interest, use of high-cost NSAIDs varied substantially based on patient characteristics. Compared with patients age 18–29, those age 30 or older were much more likely to be prescribed high-cost NSAIDs. Women and officers were somewhat more likely to be prescribed these medications, compared with men or enlisted personnel, respectively.

REFERENCES

AMEDD, *Low Back Pain Guideline Toolkit,* 1999, www.armymedicine.army.mil/.

Bero, L. A., R. Grilli, J. M. Grimshaw, E. Harvey, A. D. Oxman, and M. A. Thomson, "Closing the Gap Between Research and Practice: An Overview of Systematic Reviews of Interventions to Promote the Implementation of Research Findings," The Cochrane Effective Practice and Organization of Care Review Group, *British Medical Journal,* Vol. 317, 1998, pp. 465–468.

Cherkin, D. C., K. J. Wheeler, W. Barlow, and R. A. Deyo, "Medication Use for Low Back Pain in Primary Care," *Spine,* Vol. 23, No. 5, 1998, pp. 607–614.

Chodoff, P., and K. Crowley, "Clinical Practice Guidelines: Roadblocks to Their Acceptance and Implementation," *Journal of Outcomes Management,* Vol. 2, 1995, pp. 5–10.

Eastwood, A. J., and T. A. Sheldon, "Organisation of Asthma Care: What Difference Does It Make? A Systematic Review of the Literature," *Quality and Safety in Health Care,* Vol. 5, 1996, pp. 134–143.

Evans, R. S., S. L. Pestotnik, D. C. Classen, et al., "A Computer-Assisted Management Program for Antibiotics and Other Anti-infective Agents, *New England Journal of Medicine,* Vol. 338, 1998, pp. 232–238.

Grilli, R., and J. Lomas, "Evaluating the Message: The Relationship Between Compliance Rate and the Subject of a Practice Guideline," *Medical Care,* Vol. 32, 1994, pp. 202–213.

Grol, R., J. Dalhuijsen, S. Thomas, C. Veld, G. Rutten, and H. Mokkink, "Attributes of Clinical Guidelines That Influence Use of Guidelines in General Practice: Observational Study," *British Medical Journal,* Vol. 317, 1998, pp. 858–861.

Hargraves, J. L., R. H. Palmer, E. J. Orav, and E. A. Wright, "Practice Characteristics and Performance of Primary Care Practitioners," *Medical Care,* Vol. 34, 1996, pp. SS67–SS76.

Nicholas, W., D. Farley, M. E. Vaiana, and S. Cretin, *Putting Practice Guidelines to Work in the Department of Defense Medical System: A Guide for Action,* Santa Monica, Calif.: RAND Corporation, MR-1267-A, 2001.

Senge, P. M., *The Fifth Discipline: The Art and Practice of the Learning Organization,* New York: Doubleday/Currency, 1990.

Shortell, S. M., C. L. Bennett, and G. R. Byck, "Assessing the Impact of Continuous Quality Improvement on Clinical Practice: What It Will Take to Accelerate Progress, *Milbank Quarterly,* Vol. 76, 1998, pp. 510, 593–624.

Veterans Health Administration and Department of Defense (VHA/DoD), *VHA/DOD Clinical Practice Guideline for the Management of Low Back Pain or Sciatica in the Primary Care Setting,* Version 1.0, May 1999.

Von Korff, M., J. Gruman, J. Schaefer, S. J. Curry, and E. H. Wagner, "Collaborative Management of Chronic Illness," *Annals of Internal Medicine,* Vol. 127, 1997, pp. 1097–1102.

Wagner, E. H., B. T. Austin, and M. Von Korff, "Organizing Care for Patients with Chronic Illness," *Milbank Quarterly,* Vol. 74, 1996, pp. 511–544.